IAPSM

Case-Based Learning in COMMUNITY MEDICINE

Competency Based Training for Undergraduate and Postgraduate Students of Community Medicine

As per CBME Guidelines/Competency Based Curriculum prescribed by National Medical Commission

IAPSM
Case-Based Learning in COMMUNITY MEDICINE

Competency Based Training for Undergraduate and Postgraduate Students of Community Medicine

As per CBME Guidelines/Competency Based Curriculum prescribed by National Medical Commission

Concept and Vision

AM Kadri MBBS MD (PSM)
IAPSM National President (2023–24)

Editor-in-Chief

Purushottam Giri MBBS MD (PSM) FIAPSM MIPHA CCEBDM
Professor and Head, Department of Community Medicine
Indian Institute of Medical Science and Research
Medical College, Badnapur, Distt. Jalna, Maharashtra, India
Secretary General, IAPSM (2022–25)

Editors

Dewesh Kumar MBBS MD
Associate Professor
Department of Preventive and Social Medicine
Rajendra Institute of Medical Sciences
Ranchi, Jharkhand, India

Medha Mathur MBBS MD FAIMER
Associate Professor
Department of Community Medicine
Geetanjali Medical College and Hospital
Udaipur, Rajasthan, India

Rishabh Kumar Rana MBBS MD FPHS
Assistant Professor
Department of Community Medicine
Shaheed Nirmal Mahto Medical College
Dhanbad, Jharkhand, India

Dhruvendra Pandey MBBS MD PGDEPI
Associate Professor
Department of Community Medicine
Government Medical College
Ratlam, Madhya Pradesh, India

Advisor

Shalini Sunderam MBBS MD
Professor, Department of Community Medicine
Rajendra Institute of Medical Sciences
Ranchi, Jharkhand, India

Foreword

Sanjay Zodpey

CBSPD

CBS Publishers & Distributors Pvt Ltd

New Delhi • Bengaluru • Chennai • Kochi • Kolkata • Lucknow • Mumbai
Hyderabad • Jharkhand • Nagpur • Patna • Pune • Uttarakhand

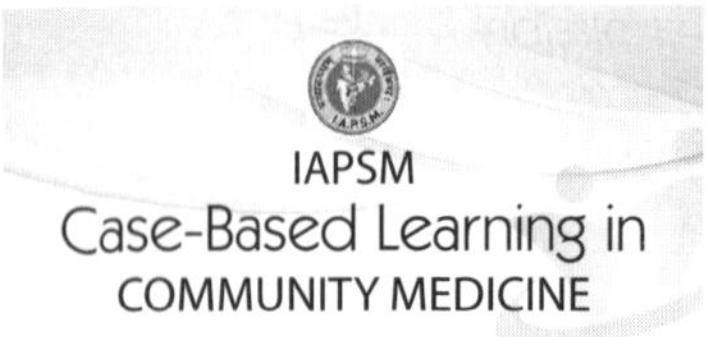

ISBN: 978-93-5466-811-1

First Edition: 2024
Reprint: 2025

Published by Satish Kumar Jain and produced by Varun Jain for

CBS Publishers & Distributors Pvt Ltd

4819/XI Prahlad Street, 24 Ansari Road, Daryaganj, New Delhi 110 002, India
Ph: 011-23266838, 23289259 Website: www.cbspd.com
e-mail: delhi@cbspd.com

Corporate Office: 204 FIE, Industrial Area, Patparganj, Delhi 110 092, India
Ph: 011-49344934 Fax: 011-49344935 e-mail: publishing@cbspd.com; publicity@cbspd.com

Branches

- **Bengaluru:** Seema House 2975, 17th Cross, K.R. Road, Banasankari 2nd Stage, Bengaluru 560 070, Karnataka, India
Ph: +91-80-26771678/79 Fax: +91-80-26771680 e-mail: bangalore@cbspd.com
- **Chennai:** 18/8B, Subbaraya Street, Shenoy Nagar, Chennai 600 030, Tamil Nadu, India
Ph: +91-44-42032115, 26681266 e-mail: chennai@cbspd.com
- **Kochi:** 42/1325, 1326, Power House Road, Opposite KSEB, Power House, Ernakulum 682018, Kochi, Kerala, India
Ph: +91-484-4059061–65 Fax: +91-484-4059065 e-mail: kochi@cbspd.com
- **Kolkata:** 147, Hind Ceramics Compound, 1st Floor, Nilgunj Road, Belghoria, Kolkata 700056, West Bengal, India
Ph: +91-33-25330055/56 e-mail: kolkata@cbspd.com
- **Lucknow:** Basement, Khushuma Complex, 7 Meerabai Marg (behind Jawahar Bhawan), Lucknow 226001, UP, India
Ph: +91-522-4000032 e-mail: tiwari.lucknow@cbspd.com
- **Mumbai:** PWD Shed, Gala No. 25/26, Ramchandra Bhatt Marg, Next JJ Hospital, Gate No. 2, Opp. Union Bank of India, Noorbaug Mumbai 400009, Maharashtra, India
Ph: +91-22-66661880/89 e-mail: mumbai@cbspd.com

Representatives

- **Hyderabad** 0-9885175004
- **Jharkhand** 0-9811541605
- **Nagpur** 0-8692091830
- **Patna** 0-9334159340
- **Pune** 0-9664372571
- **Uttarakhand** 0-9716462459

Printed at: Rashtriya Printer, Dilshad Garden, Delhi

to

---

all past Presidents and
past Secretary Generals
who nurtured
IAPSM to reach this level

Reviewers

Dr Deepak Saxena *MBBS MD (PSM)*	***Dr Gajanan Velhal*** *MBBS MD (PSM)*	***Dr Pradeep Deshmukh*** *MBBS MD (PSM)*
Director Indian Institute of Public Health (IIPH) Gandhinagar, Gujarat	Professor and Head Department of Community Medicine Seth GS Medical College and KEM Hospital, Mumbai, Maharashtra	Professor and Head Department of Community Medicine and Family Medicine AIIMS, Nagpur, Maharashtra

Contributors

Ajeet Singh Bhadoria
Department of Community Medicine, and Family Medicine
AIIMS, Rishikesh, Uttarakhand

Anit Kujur
Department of PSM
RIMS, Ranchi, Jharkhand

Ayush Lohia
Department of Public Health
Kalyan Singh Super Specialty Cancer Institute
Lucknow, UP

Chandramani Kumar
Department of Community Medicine
SBMC, Hazaribagh, Jharkhand

Deepti Dabar
Department of Community and Family Medicine
AIIMS, Bhopal, MP

Dewesh Kumar
Department of PSM
RIMS, Ranchi, Jharkhand

Dhruvendra Pandey
Department of Community Medicine
Government Medical College
Ratlam, MP

Kanchan Gawande
Department of Community Medicine, and Family Medicine
AIIMS, Rishikesh, Uttarakhand

Krupal Joshi
Department of Community and Family Medicine
AIIMS, Rajkot, Gujarat

Medha Mathur
Department of Community Medicine
GMCH, Udaipur, Rajasthan

Nazish Rasheed
Department of Community Medicine
LHMC, New Delhi

Nilanjana Ghosh
Department of Community and Family Medicine
AIIMS, Guwahati, Assam

Nisha Murmu
Department of Community and Family Medicine
AIIMS, Bhubaneshwar, Odisha

Nitesh Kumar
Department of Community and Family Medicine
AIIMS, Jammu

Nitika Keshri
Department of PSM
RIMS, Ranchi, Jharkhand

Purushottam Giri
Department of Community Medicine
IIMSR Medical College, Jalna, Maharashtra

Rama Shankar Rath
Department of Community and Family Medicine
AIIMS, Gorakhpur, UP

Rishabh Kumar Rana
Department of PSM
SNMMC, Dhanbad, Jharkhand

Sanjeet Panesar
Department of Community Medicine
ABVIMS and RML Hospital, New Delhi

Sanjeev Kumar
Department of Community and Family Medicine
AIIMS, Bhopal, MP

Setu Sinha
Department of Community Medicine
IGIMS, Patna, Bihar

Shashi Bhushan Singh
Department of PSM
RIMS, Ranchi, Jharkhand

Soumitra Sethia
Department of Community Medicine
Government Medical College
Khandwa, MP

Tulika Singh
Department of Community Medicine
IGIMS, Patna, Bihar

Venkatashiva Reddy B
Department of Community and Family Medicine
AIIMS, Manglagiri, AP

Vikas Yadav
Department of Environmental Health and Epidemiology
ICMR-NIREH, Bhopal, MP

Foreword

The public health system plays a vital role in the well-being of every country. Since decades, the role of community medicine is pivotal in practicing preventive, curative, and holistic strategies for good health of the population. The importance of the fundamental principles of preventive medicine should be made clear among undergraduate and postgraduate students. Indian Association of Preventive and Social Medicine (IAPSM) encourages its members to create resource materials for generating efficient workforce to handle real world challenges in the form of diseases and health-related events.

Medical schools and departments of community medicine are particularly instrumental in training the next generation of mystically and socially relevant health professionals. The training in community medicine for the undergraduate students equips these young professionals with a taste of real-life mutations within the Indian health system. Postgraduate students take a deep dive into the practice of the subject. All these professional undergraduates as well as postgraduates will be at the front lines of our health system in the years to come. They need the right competencies to handle any situation posed to them. For better understanding and practice of these competencies, it is important to tickle the higher cognitive domain of the students. Keeping this thing in mind, the book, *Case-Based Learning in Community Medicine,* has been compiled which emphasizes skill acquisition and the ability to apply the knowledge gained to practical situations. The book is unique in a manner that it provides hundreds of case scenario-based questions for practice. The book covers all the important topics of community medicine curriculum and helps the health professionals to decipher scenario-based public health problems and discuss solutions to respond to those problems. The reviewers and advisors have inculcated their experiences in the book to meet the competency-based learning in community medicine.

Sanjay Zodpey
President
Public Health Foundation of India (PHFI), New Delhi

Prologue

I have noted Western world making learning so interesting, and the teachers generate a sense of interest amongst the students for the subjects. They apply all the new methods of teaching in classroom to make every student engaged and understand the importance of the topic and subject. One of these methods, which our National Medical Commission suggests, is case-based learning (CBL). Case-based learning in our subject will certainly generate more interest than giving lectures through AV aids. Even the assessment pattern also has questions based on CBL to evaluate the learning of the student. Although there are many teachers who teach various topics applying this principle but most of our budding teachers do not have idea about this type of learning. So, this book will provide a guide to the teachers as well as students to have the deep understanding of the topics of our subject. This is the first book of its kind in the field of community medicine and will pave a way to new learning approaches to medical teachers. After the IAPSM textbook, I thought of CBL book and I asked a few of the young IAPSM members to conceptualize and work upon it. I am happy to announce that under the leadership of Prof Dr Purushottam Giri, Secretary General of IAPSM, this book is a reality now and soon will be available for us and our students to connect more with the real case-based situations in community.

AM Kadri
President
Indian Association of Preventive and
Social Medicine (IAPSM) (2023–24)

Preface

The purpose of writing this book is to provide medical undergraduates and postgraduates with an understanding of competency-based medical education and broaden their thinking through case-based learning (CBL). It seeks to move away from traditional methods of teaching, while providing valid references from recognized books at the same time. It is designed to equip the learners with the necessary skills and knowledge to provide care effectively and efficiently in the community setting. The well-curated exercises shall encourage the reader to think critically and apply the knowledge they have gained to real world scenarios.

The community medicine physicians from all over the country were approached and a team of enthusiast physicians came forward to put their individual effort towards this book. Each chapter is written by an expert in the field, who shares his insights and experiences, and provides practical guidance on how to set about each case. This approach via CBL could be effective in improving the field experiences of healthcare providers, particularly in identifying and managing ill health and serving as a first point of contact for any health issues within the community. It will encourage the development of analytical skills as well as the necessary skill to develop interpersonal relations, and the application of evidence-based practices to improve standard of care, ultimately leading to better outcomes for patients.

It is also hoped that this approach will give a deeper understanding of the complexities of the healthcare system and the challenges faced by patients, hence urging the reader to be forward-thinking yet persevering. This book is the result of collective efforts of many experts in the field of community medicine from all over the country. I personally thank each and every faculty for giving a lot of efforts in such a short period of time and coming out with such a comprehensive book. Definitely, there is a scope of improvement. So we all are eager to have your valuable feedback and suggestions for improving this book in subsequent editions.

Purushottam Giri
Editor-in-Chief

Contents

Case Exercises with Respective Competencies

Sr. No.	Chapter	No. of Case Exercises	Page No.	Competencies
1.	Family and Community Health	10	1	CM2.1, CM2.2, CM2.4, CM2.5, CM3.1, CM3.4, CM5.2, CM5.3, CM5.4, CM8.1, CM10.3, CM10.6, CM12.1, CM12.3, PH1.55
2.	Environmental Health	19	9	CM3.1, CM3.2, CM3.5, CM8.1, CM8.3, CM8.4, CM8.7, CM9.1, CM10.5, MI8.16, PA12.1, PH1.55
3.	Epidemiology	20	20	CM7.3, CM7.4, CM7.7, CM9.1, CM9.2, CM10.1, CM12.1, PH1.55
4.	Research Methodology	19	29	CM3.2, CM6.1, CM6.2, CM6.3, CM7.1, CM7.3, CM7.5, CM7.6, CM7.8, CM14.1, CM14.2
5.	Biostatistics	19	37	CM6.1, CM6.2, CM6.3, CM6.4, CM7.1, CM7.5, CM7.8, CM7.9, CM9.1, CM9.4, PH1.55
6.	Health Communication	11	49	CM1.4, CM1.5, CM1.6, CM1.9, CM1.10, CM2.3, CM4.1, CM4.2, CM6.2, IM4.3, MI8.6, MI8.7
7.	Immunization	22	55	CM7.2, CM7.9, CM8.1, CM8.3, CM8.4, CM8.5, CM8.6, CM10.5, CM10.8, CM17.3, CM17.5, CM19.1, CM20.2, CT1.1, CT1.15, CT1.16, CT1.18, IM4.3, IM9.15, IM25.1, IM25.13, MI1.3, MI8.4, MI8.16, OG1.2, OG8.1, OG19.2, OG33.3, PE3.5, PE9.1, PE9.2, PE9.7, PE10.4, PE17.1, PE17.2, PE18.1, PE18.2, PE18.3, PE18.6, PE18.8, PE19.1, PE19.2, PE19.3, PE19.4, PE19.5, PE19.12, PE29.5, PH1.55
8.	Infectious Diseases	18	71	CM1.5, CM3.3, CM5.3, CM7.7, CM8.1, CM8.3, CM8.5, CM10.5, CM20.2, IM4.3, MI1.3, MI8.4, PE3.5, PE3.7, PE8.1, PE8.2, PE8.3, PE8.4, PE8.5, PE9.1, PE9.2, PE9.5, PE9.6, PE10.4, PE17.1, PE19.1 PE19.2, PE19.3, PE19.4, PE19.5, PH1.55
9.	Non-Communicable Diseases	10	83	CM2.2, CM2.4, CM2.5, CM8.2, CM15.3, PS19.1, PS19.2
10.	Nutrition	20	88	CM5.1, CM5.2, CM5.3, CM5.5, CM5.7, CM5.8, CM10.3, IM9.15, PE8.1, PE8.2
11.	Maternal and Child Health	21	98	CM10.1, CM10.2, CM10.3, CM10.4, CM10.5, CM10.6, CM10.7, CM10.8, OG1.1
12.	Family Planning	12	109	CM9.4, CM9.5, CM9.6, CM10.6, CM10.7, OG21.1

Contd...

Contd...

CHAPTER 1

Family and Community Health

Competency code	Competency addressed	Exercise
CM2.1	Describe the steps and perform clinico-socio-cultural and demographic assessment of the individual, family and community	1.1
CM2.2	Describe the socio-cultural factors, family (types), its role in health and disease & demonstrate in a simulated environment the correct assessment of socio-economic status	1.3
CM2.4	Describe social psychology, community behavior and community relationship and their impact on health and disease	1.6
CM2.5	Describe poverty and social security measures and its relationship to health and disease	1.7
CM3.1	Describe the health hazards of air, water, noise, radiation and pollution	1.3
CM3.4	Describe the concept of solid waste, human excreta and sewage disposal	1.3
CM5.2	Describe and demonstrate the correct method of performing a nutritional assessment of individuals, families and the community by using the appropriate method	1.8
CM5.3	Define and describe common nutrition related health disorders (including macro-PEM, Micro-iron, Zn, iodine, Vit. A), their control and management	1.2
CM5.4	Plan and recommend a suitable diet for the individuals and families based on local availability of foods and economic status, etc. in a simulated environment	1.2
CM8.1	Describe and discuss the epidemiological and control measures including the use of essential laboratory tests at the primary care level for communicable diseases	1.10
CM10.3	Describe local customs and practices during pregnancy, childbirth, lactation and child feeding practices	1.4
CM10.6	Enumerate and describe various family planning methods, their advantages and shortcomings	1.5
CM12.1	Define and describe the concept of geriatric services	1.9
CM12.3	Describe the prevention of health problems of aged population	1.9
PH1.55	Describe and discuss the following National Health programs including Immunization, Tuberculosis, Leprosy, Malaria, HIV, Filaria, Kala azar, Diarrheal diseases, Anemia & nutritional disorders, Blindness, Non-communicable diseases, Cancer and Iodine deficiency	1.10

Guide Notes

- Different socio-economic status (SES) classification scales used in India and elsewhere
- Sewage disposal
- Water and sanitation.

EXERCISE 1.4

At the end of this exercise, you should be able to describe local customs and practices during pregnancy, childbirth, lactation and child feeding practices **(CM10.3)**

The index case is a 21-year-old lactating mother with her 17-day old neonate. She is a $P_1L_1A_0$ (obstetric history) who delivered through cesarean section on July 12, 2020. She is presented with symptoms of heartburn and pain at the stitch site for past 2 days. There is a negative history of fever, lower abdominal pain, copious or offensive lochia discharge, itching, bleeding p/v, burning micturition, nausea, regurgitation, or pain in breasts after delivery. She had her menarche at 14 years of age. Her cycles have by far been regular and there were no complaints of dysmenorrhea or menorrhagia. Her last menstrual period (LMP) and expected date of delivery (EDD) were October 2, 2019 and July 9, 2020, respectively. Initially she was unaware of her pregnancy and complained of morning sickness, nausea, vomiting and fatigue in the first trimester. Pregnancy was confirmed by urine pregnancy test (UPT) in the 3rd month by a private practitioner, after which she got herself registered at RIMS, Ranchi. Ultrasonography (TAS/TVS) was done during her antenatal visits to the hospital. She took iron-folic acid (IFA) regularly and received 2 doses of tetanus (TT) vaccination. She reported quickening in the fourth gestational month. Her weight at full term was 55 kg and Hb was measured to be 11.6 g/dl. She had to undergo an elective caesarean section due to mal-presentation. The baby cried soon after birth and weighed 2.75 kg. The baby was breastfed after 12 hours of birth and received birth doses of the following vaccines: BCG, OPV and Hep B. The baby was not bathed for the first 4 days. The mother and the baby were discharged after 4 days. Currently, the mother is breastfeeding the baby as and when she cries, approximately about 6–7 times in the day and 2–3 times at night. In between, the mother also feeds the baby with gripe water when she cries in the evening as per the family's suggestion. The mother is not a Janani Suraksha Yojana (JSY) beneficiary. She is a non-vegetarian by diet. Based on 24-hour recall method, she had 1 glass of milk, 2 tsp sugar, 1 *Panjiri laddoo* (1 serving amounts to 464 calories), 12 *rotis*, 1 *katori aloo palak sabzi* and 1 *katori bhindi sabzi*. The mother's current weight is 42 kg and height is 150 cm. The baby and the mother, altogether appear normal on general examination.

- What wrong practices can you point out in the above scenario? What ideally should be practiced instead?
- Comment on the ANC care of the mother and weight and immunization of the baby at birth?

Guide Notes

- Recommendations by WHO for ANC and PNC visits and that for Indian scenario.

EXERCISE 1.5

At the end of this exercise, you should be able to enumerate and describe various family planning methods, their advantages and shortcomings **(CM10.6)**

During the induction visit under Family Adoption Programme, you come across a family constituting of 6 members. The head of family (HOF), Sanjay, is a 32 years old male, with no formal education, and earns a living by selling fruits in the local market. The wife of the HOF is a 27 years old female Radhika, who is a homemaker. The other 4 members are three daughters and one son, including a newborn; the eldest among them being a 5 years and 6 months old daughter, Neha. Neha caught your attention, since you noticed grossly visible deformity in both her legs, which the mother had noticed when Neha was 2 years old.

- Prepare a case presentation having two parts:
  - The first part should describe the family's composition, physical and biological environment, dietary history, socio-cultural environment, ending in a family diagnosis of the apparent needs of this family.
  - The second part of the presentation should be a case study taking Neha as the index case, which should also include antenatal, intra-natal and postnatal history when Radhika conceived her.

  (For preparing the presentation, you might have to interact with various families and assimilate information in this single presentation.)
- Also highlight the advice you think is appropriate in this scenario, general for family and specific to Neha.

Guide Notes

- Objectives of family study
- Family Adoption Programme
- Various models for FAP and which one is followed by your institute.

EXERCISE 1.6

At the end of this exercise, you should be able to describe social psychology, community behaviour and community relationship and their impact on health and disease **(CM2.4)**

You adopt a six-membered, Hindu, non-vegetarian, upper lower-class family residing in their own house in Dallapura. The head of the family (HOF) is a 45 years old male, Gopal, with formal education till 8th class and working under a contractor. He is a chronic alcoholic and smoker. His wife, Vijaywati, 41 years old, is illiterate and works in a factory as a daily-wage labourer. They have 4 children, the eldest being 23 years old Sonu, their only son, who also works in the same factory as his mother. Sonu has attained formal education till 6th class only. Two out of 3 daughters dropped out from school after completing their 3rd standard education, whilst the youngest is in the 3rd standard currently. A distressed Sonu called you one night informing you about his mothers' ill health. Vijaywati is having difficulty in breathing and looks pale and drowsy, as she has been crying on the floor for the past one hour. Sonu heard loud voices coming from his parents' room, as if they were fighting. He also mentions some bruise marks on her face and arm, and pain in right ankle. On further enquiry, Sonu informs you that she had fever, cough with yellowish sputum production and chest pain for the last 4–5 days. She also complained of heartburn and weakness for the past one month. Apprehending a case of domestic violence (DV), you ask Sonu to bring his mother to the hospital immediately.

- Draft a case presentation in two parts: Generalized Family Structure and case of Domestic Violence as the index.

- What preliminary questions would you ask Sonu over the call to assess Vijaywati's condition?
- What other measures would you want Sonu to take before leaving for hospital?
- Explain "Right to Health for All" in context of Indian women.

Guide Notes

- Health issues associated with DV
- Impact of DV on children (physical health and mental health) in the family
- Judiciary and community help in cases of DV and sexual assault (SA).

EXERCISE 1.7

At the end of this exercise, you should be able to describe poverty and social security measures and its relationship to health and disease **(CM2.5)**

During your first visit, you had to analyze the socio-economic status (SES) of the family in the above exercise.

Parameter	***Status***
Education of Head of the family (HOF)	8th Pass
Occupation of HOF	Semi-skilled
Family income per month	₹ 8500/-

- Using Kuppuswamy classification scale, determine the SES of the family.
- Also classify according to Modified BG Prasad SES scale?

Guide Notes

- Tendulkar Committee
- Various SES scales
- BPL card and health benefits
- Availing benefits under AB.

EXERCISE 1.8

At the end of this exercise, you should be able to describe and demonstrate the correct method of performing a nutritional assessment of individuals, families and the community by using the appropriate method **(CM5.2)**

You examine an 11 years old, Pooja, student of 5th class section B, of Nagar Nigam Prathmik Balika Vidyalaya, Shahdara, Delhi. She resides in Kheda region with her family comprising her father (driver), mother (housewife), elder brother Mohan (13 years old, studies in 7th standard) and younger sister Sandhya (3 years old, stays at home). Sandhya was delivered prematurely at 33 weeks, other than that there is no significant past history. Her height and weight are 143 cm and 25 kg, respectively. She has an average built. Her skin appears normal, with no apparent edema, rash, or pigmentary issues. Her hair seems lustrous. Grossly, her eye, ENT and oral examinations were insignificant. Lymph nodes were not palpable and no apparent swelling which moved with deglutition was present in front of the neck. Systemic examination was done, which only revealed a 6/9 vision with spectacles, bilaterally. She mentioned that she eats food prepared at home only, but still experiences frequent stomach aches, gastrointestinal (GI) upset, flatulence, and occasional loose motions. There was no record of vaccination since birth.

- What is the structure of a School Health Card?
- Draft one for Pooja with duly filled information.

Guide Notes

- Structure of Family Card and School Heath Card
- Structure of Nutritional Assessment Survey Form
- Locally available combination food with their nutritive values and recommended daily intake, as per different age groups
- Emerging GI issues and the appropriate dietary adjustments.

EXERCISE 1.9

- At the end of this exercise, you should be able to define and describe the concept of Geriatric services **(CM12.1)**
- Describe the prevention of health problems of aged population **(CM12.3)**

Study the following family composition:

S. No.	Name	Age/Sex	Relation to HOF	Literacy	Occupation
1.	Rani Devi	62/F	Mother	5th pass	–
2.	Arvind	40/M	Self	12th pass	Auto driver
3.	Rekha	35/F	Wife	8th pass	Housewife
4.	Siddhant	9/M	Son	4th class	Student in Government school
5.	Sneha	7/F	Daughter	2nd class	Student in Government school

Rani Devi was apparently well 7 years back when she complained of insidious onset of increased frequency and burning micturition. A few days later she developed high grade fever and was brought to GTB hospital emergency in an unconscious state, where she was diagnosed with diabetes and hypertension. She was started on treatment at the GTB hospital, but she was non-compliant to her medications. She used to get her blood sugar tested at regular intervals of 3–6 months. Recently she has started to complain about chest pain on left side which radiated to jaws and epigastric region. The pain is dull in nature, intermittent and associated with gradually worsening dyspnea. She complains about blurring of vision and seeing floating objects in her visual field.

- What advice will you give to Arvind and Rekha as the caretaker of Rani Devi, regarding her care?
- Make two groups, each having four people, who will educate the whole class about the following four topics related to diabetes and hypertension.
    - Signs and symptoms
    - Investigations and follow-up visits
    - Management protocol, with proper dosing of medicines
    - Dangers signs, complications, and their management.

Guide Notes

- BP Passport, IHCI
- Geriatric care and jurisprudence.

EXERCISE 1.10

- At the end of this exercise, you should be able to describe and discuss the following National Health programs including Immunization, Tuberculosis, Leprosy, Malaria, HIV, Filaria, Kala azar, Diarrheal diseases, Anemia and nutritional disorders, Blindness, Non-communicable diseases, Cancer and lodine deficiency **(PH1.55)**
- Describe and discuss the epidemiological and control measures including the use of essential laboratory tests at the primary care level for communicable diseases **(CM8.1)**

Vipin, a 32 years old male who is a known case of tuberculosis, is adherent to his treatment plan and is about to complete the continuation phase in 15 days. He presents to the community health centre (CHC) with his wife Manjiri, 26 years old, with complains of irregular menses and scanty bleeding per cycle, since 6 months. She also has evening rise of temperature and increased coughing since 8 months, with mild sputum production occasionally. The couple is not practicing any contraception and has been married for 14 months. Her last cycle was delayed by two weeks, so she went to the nearby primary health care (PHC) and was advised to take up a urine pregnancy test, which subsequently came out to be negative. Since the couple is planning for a baby, the doctor had prescribed her IFA tablets and advised her to get a USG pelvis done. She did not get the ultrasound done, as she had her menses in a couple of days. On eliciting past medical history, she informs that she had not been vaccinated with her birth doses and received her first vaccine at the age of 2 years. She also had contracted TB from her father at the age of 15 years but is not sure whether she completed the treatment or not. She also did not go for follow up testing then. You advise her USG pelvis and sputum examination for acid fast bacilli (AFB) and computer based nucleic acid amplification test (CBNAAT).

- What is your provisional diagnosis of Manjiri's condition?
- Discuss among yourselves the need and scope of premarital counselling and screening for communicable and non-communicable diseases.

Guide Notes

- DOTS centre in your area
- Complications of TB and danger signs.

REFERENCES

1. Kadri's IAPSM's Textbook of Community Medicine. 2nd edn, pages 66, 68, 893, 643, 594, 962
2. Park's Textbook of Preventive and Social Medicine. 26th edn, Chapters-14 'Tribal Health in India', and Chapter-24 'Health Care of the Community'.

CHAPTER 2

Environmental Health

Competency code	Competency addressed	Exercise
CM3.1	Describe the health hazards of air, water, noise, radiation and pollution	2.1, 2.2, 2.5–2.9, 2.14, 2,15, 2,18
CM3.2	Describe concepts of safe and wholesome water, sanitary sources of water, water purification processes, water quality standards, concepts of water conservation and rainwater harvesting	2.4, 2.19
CM3.5	Describe the standards of housing and the effect of housing on Health	2.4
CM8.1	Describe and discuss the epidemiological and control measures including the use of essential laboratory tests at the primary care level for communicable diseases	2.10
CM8.3	Enumerate and describe disease specific National Health Programs including their prevention and treatment of a case	2.13
CM8.4	Describe the principles and enumerate the measures to control a disease epidemic	2.10, 2.16
CM8.7	Describe the principles of management of information systems	2.12
CM9.1	Define and describe the principles of demography, demographic cycle, vital statistics	2.17
CM10.5	Describe Universal Immunization Program; Integrated Management of Neonatal and Childhood Illness (IMNCI) and other existing Programs	2.2, 2.3
MI8.16	Describe the National Health Programs in the prevention of common infectious disease.	2.11
PA12.1	Enumerate and describe the pathogenesis of disorders caused by air pollution, tobacco and alcohol	2.5
PH1.55	Describe and discuss the following national health programs including Immunization, Tuberculosis, Leprosy, Malaria, HIV, Filaria, Kala Azar, Diarrheal diseases, Anemia and nutritional disorders, Blindness, Non-communicable diseases, Cancer and Iodine deficiency.	2.11

The funnel for receiving the rainfall has a diameter of 5 inches. Great care is exercised in selecting a suitable site for the erection of rain-gauge. The rain-gauge should be set on a level ground, away from trees, buildings, or other obstructions. Used by farmers and the Meteorological Department, it is an important tool for collecting data regarding rainfall.

- What are the other names for this instrument?
- Enlist the common problems encountered while taking readings using this device?
- Mention the accuracy and measurement units of this device?

Guide Notes

- Types of rain gauges
- Rain gauge used in India.

EXERCISE 2.5

- At the end of this exercise, you should be able to describe the health hazards of air, water, noise, radiation and pollution **(CM3.1)**
- Enumerate and describe the pathogenesis of disorders caused by air pollution, tobacco and alcohol **(PA12.1)**

During one Lok Sabha session, a MP asked the minister of the concerned ministry about the maximum permissible levels of the airborne particulate matter (PM), its types and the effect which the extension of range will have on checking air pollution.

- Which ministry of GoI concerns itself with air quality and pollution?
- Posted under that Ministry you were asked by the Principal Secretary to give the details of various airborne particulate matter (PM) with its normal range of permissible limits. Can you mention those?
- How can the said range extension help in controlling air pollution?
- Enumerate the various other pollutants listed by CPCB along with their permissible limits.

Guide Notes

- Central Pollution Control Board
- Ambient Air Quality Standards, India.

EXERCISE 2.6

At the end of this exercise, you should be able to describe the health hazards of air, water, noise, radiation and pollution **(CM3.1)**

Climate change and its effect on health are often debated and has evoked arguments, both favoring as well as denying the situation. For example, an Archbishop of Sydney criticized the concept of climate change and subsequently a need to cut down on 'Green House emissions', the other being former US President calling the idea of global warming a hoax.

- What challenges do you expect to face as a public health expert/doctor while convincing the public about the health concerns related to global warming and their participation for its resolution?
- Suggest some actionable points based on your current understanding of the topic.

Guide Notes

- Recent updates about climate change
- Discuss the various arguments given by both those who do and those who do not think climate change is concerning.

EXERCISE 2.7

At the end of this exercise, you should be able to describe the health hazards of air, water, noise, radiation and pollution **(CM3.1)**

Air Quality Index (AQI) is an important tool as it can conveniently convey to the common public about the quality of the ambient air which helps them better adapt and prepare to safeguard themselves from the hazards of pollution. In present days, portable devices connected to the internet can also show the AQI of the region the person has travelled to. Observed values of various pollutants help in calculating the AQI.

- Which pollutants are considered for calculation of AQI?
- Mention the various categories based on levels of AQI.
- What are health breakpoints in calculation of AQI?

Guide Note

- Indoor AQI (IAQI) and Thermal Comfort Index (TCI).

EXERCISE 2.8

At the end of this exercise, you should be able to describe the health hazards of air, water, noise, radiation and pollution **(CM3.1)**

While watching advertisements for a car or a bike, you notice a Bharat Stage sticker on the vehicle which was being highlighted during the advertisement. In India, it is done by a separate Ministry. These staging and associated regulations can even be attributed to phasing out the 2-stroke engines for two wheelers and extinction of Maruti 800 cc cars. Two committees were set up in 2002 and 2012, respectively, whose reports paved the way to bring about these changes. The committees sequentially proposed roadmaps for the steps needed to ensure healthier and cleaner air.

- Mention the various Bharat Stages along with the year in which they were introduced.
- Name the ministry/ministries involved in these regulations, changes, and their execution across the country.
- Name the committees and their salient features which brought about a paradigm shift in the way environment is taken care of without active participation.

Guide Notes

- BSES
- Mashelkar Committee
- Expert Committee under Saumitra Chaudhuri

EXERCISE 2.9

At the end of this exercise, you should be able to describe the health hazards of air, water, noise, radiation and pollution **(CM3.1)**

Carbon monoxide (CO) is one of the most common air pollutants. Usually produced due to incomplete combustion of the fuel either from automobiles, coal, wood, timber, heating facilities, incinerators or any carbon containing material. As we know, hemoglobin has a greater affinity for CO as compared to oxygen, hence it causes toxicity which can be fatal if not diagnosed and treated on time.

- Discuss ill-effects of CO inhalation in both healthy people, and people with any preexisting morbidity.
- Enlist the pollutants present along with CO and how their levels are affected when CO emissions are controlled?
- What is meant by an 8-hour exposure limit for carbon monoxide?

Guide Notes

- OSHA standards for CO exposure
- Carbon monoxide poisoning (acute and chronic).

EXERCISE 2.10

- At the end of this exercise, you should be able to describe and discuss the epidemiological and control measures including the use of essential laboratory tests at the primary care level for communicable diseases **(CM8.1)**
- Describe the principles and enumerate the measures to control a disease epidemic **(CM8.4)**

During the COVID-19 pandemic, some terms became common knowledge among the public, like 'isolation' and 'quarantine'. These terms date back to 15th century when used for diseases like Black Death, Plague, Spanish Flu, etc. Currently, they were highlighted in the media when used to denote quarantine centers or isolation centers, which were set up in both, the rural and urban areas. Dedicated COVID-19 hospitals too were developed in similar way in India and across the globe.

- Define quarantine and its importance in context of disease containment, especially infectious diseases of the respiratory tract.
- Define the term isolation and its importance in context of disease containment, especially infectious diseases of the respiratory tract.
- What is a dedicated COVID-19 hospital and the ministry which formulates the guidelines for its functioning?

Guide Note

- COVID-19: Management of cases in India.

EXERCISE 2.11

- At the end of this exercise, you should be able to describe the National Health Programs in the prevention of common infectious disease **(MI8.16)**
- Describe and discuss the following National Health programs including Immunization, Tuberculosis, Leprosy, Malaria, HIV, Filaria, Kala azar, Diarrheal diseases, Anemia and nutritional disorders, Blindness, Non-communicable diseases, Cancer and Iodine deficiency **(PH1.55)**

Pulmonary tuberculosis is an ailment which continues to burden our society and therefore the healthcare system. The battle with tuberculosis has been partly won with interventions like vaccination, newer drugs, and modified regimens. Mycobacterium tuberculi has, over time, developed resistance to treatment, evolving into MDR-TB and

XDR-TB strains. With programme like RNTCP, India too has made rapid progress in the fight against tuberculosis. In 2017, certain changes have been made to its guidelines to control and prevent transmission of TB.

- Detail out the changes (in terms of addition of drugs) to combat the resistant strains.
- What is the exact role of vaccines in tuberculosis control particularly in Indian context?
- In terms of COVID-19 pandemic, respiratory etiquette has hogged the limelight. Pan out the effects that precautions taken in COVID-19 pandemic had on TB epidemiology.

Guide Notes

- Revised National Tuberculosis Control Programme (RNTCP) and National Tuberculosis Elimination Programme (NTEP)
- National Health Policy (NHP), 2017.

EXERCISE 2.12

At the end of this exercise, you should be able to describe the principles of management of information systems **(CM8.7)**

In a Medical College and Hospital, a pregnant female aged 29 years, came to the emergency department, in the month of March 2020, complaining of difficulty in breathing, heaviness in the chest, cough, and fever more than 38°C, progressing since last two days. She was admitted in the general ward of the medicine department. After two days of her admission, similar symptoms were noted in other patients close to her bed. This prompted the authorities to separate such cases and keep their beds at least 1.5 meters apart and the treating doctors and nurses were cautioned to practice extra safety measures like repeated hand washing and wearing a mask when interacting with such patients. A detailed history of the former patient revealed that she came from a locality which is crowded and few of her family members and neighbors were having cough and fever for the last seven days, some of which have recovered.

- Based on her symptoms, classify her according to Influenza Surveillance Protocol of WHO.
- Who should have noted these symptoms and alerted the system that a potential influenza case is admitted in the general ward.
- Can you name any agency, national or international, to which such cases must be reported?

Guide Note

- WHO Influenza Surveillance.

EXERCISE 2.13

At the end of this exercise, you should be able to enumerate and describe disease specific National Health Programs including their prevention and treatment of a case **(CM8.3)**

A 45-years-old, middle-aged male presents to the OPD, with history of acute episodes of asthma, complaining of dyspnea. Presently he is maintained on steroid inhalation. He works as a shopkeeper at a general store, which is situated alongside a busy street market, and he is generally surrounded by cereal dust, dirt, and fine particulate matters, most of the days. He rarely goes out in the sun and is mostly seated indoors. He smokes 3 cigarettes a day and seldom drinks any alcohol. He has a non-vegetarian diet and has known allergy to eggs. He is non-hypertensive and non-diabetic.

- What is the public health point of view in this presentation of the individual regarding the disease?
- Can you suggest public health interventions so that the disease can be prevented from happening to other individuals?
- Can you name the programme being run by GoI which caters to such cases and tries to create awareness along with generation of data for such cases?

Guide Notes

- NPCDCS (National Programme for Prevention and Control of Cancer, Diabetes, Cardiovascular Diseases and Stroke).
- NP-NCD (National Program for Prevention of Non-communicable Diseases)

EXERCISE 2.14

At the end of this exercise, you should be able to describe the health hazards of air, water, noise, radiation and pollution **(CM3.1)**

Readers of the famous Sherlock Holmes, written by Sir Arthur Conan Doyle, must be familiar with the London fog or the fog over the river Thames in the city of London in 1800s, chronicled by him. This fog has been there since the beginning of the industrial revolution around the 1600s. However, the science behind it was not explored till the 1980s, when over the years deaths were attributed due to its ill-effects on health. Of late Delhi was also mostly highlighted in media about the fog or smog which worsened during the winters. Environmental pollution to such a level mandates urgent measures from governments of those regions, to safeguard their citizens and the environment.

- Name the act passed by the GoI to safeguard environment in India.
- Name the environment protection authorities of India.
- Can you name any surveillance body which possesses the authority to conduct surprise checks?

Guide Note

- Environment Protection Act, 1986.

EXERCISE 2.15

At the end of this exercise, you should be able to describe the health hazards of air, water, noise, radiation and pollution **(CM3.1)**

Specific absorption rate (SAR) is a measure of the rate at which energy is absorbed per unit mass by a human body when exposed to a radio frequency electromagnetic field and is expressed in watts per kilogram (W/kg). SARs are difficult to calculate and must be converted to intensity limits for enforcement. With the increasing trend of online classes, video tutorials, online tests, and meetings, which somehow mandates the use of mobile phones and tablets, one must also not forget to practice 'sleep hygiene'. As one is exposed to more mobiles and laptops, SAR plays an important role in deciding what happens due to this prolonged exposure.

- What do SAR levels warn about?
- Prior to mobile phones, do you know any other appliance being used in your home that had a SAR limit? If yes, how much was the limit?
- What is sleep hygiene and under which important aspect of sleep hygiene does keeping away mobile phones and laptops before going to bed come?
- What exactly is the average SAR of your mobile device being used and are they in confirmation to the limits set by your country?
- Can you name any long-term cohort study which tried to explore the ill effects of using prolonged mobile phones?

Guide Note

- Ensuring safety from Radiations: Mobile towers and Handsets, Department of Telecommunication, Government of India.

EXERCISE 2.16

At the end of this exercise, you should be able to describe the principles and enumerate the measures to control a disease epidemic **(CM8.4)**

When the COVID-19 pandemic struck India and the first case was reported on January 30, 2020. However, as the cases started increasing, GoI took major steps a mock 'Lockdown 'under the name of "Junta Curfew" was initiated by Prime Minister Shree Narendra Modi on March 21, 2020, where in all citizens were requested not to leave their houses except those involved in indispensable emergency services. Following which immediately on March 22 the entire Nation was ushered into a Lockdown, along with which an old act, known as the Epidemic Disease Act, was revoked.

- When the Epidemic Disease Act was originally enacted in India?
- What changes/amendments were made in the Epidemic Disease Act when it was reenacted during the COVID-19 crisis in India?
- Mention the conditions under which the Act can be applied.

Guide Notes

- Epidemic Disease Act, 1897
- Epidemic Diseases (Amendment) Ordinance, 2020.

EXERCISE 2.17

At the end of this exercise, you should be able to define and describe the principles of Demography, Demographic cycle, vital statistics **(CM9.1)**

Migration and displacement have always been features of human life but the intensification of globalization, and increased ease of travel and interconnectedness has seen the effects of displacement reaching far beyond the immediate contexts in which they occur. Forced migration is displacement that involves coercion and the implication that those involved have moved against their will. In the previous few decades with the end of the cold war, rapid globalization, increasing inequality between and within nations, ongoing wars, climate change and conflict [United Nations High Commissioner for Refugees (UNHCR) 2006 report], a landscape has been created where forced migration affects all populations to some extent, whether they are the displaced themselves or are hosts to the displaced.

- Define forced migration and name the organization which has given the definition.
- Categorize the various accepted types of forced migration.

Guide Note

- Effect of migration on population dynamics.

EXERCISE 2.18

At the end of this exercise, you should be able to describe the health hazards of air, water, noise, radiation and pollution **(CM3.1)**

The famous cricketer Mr. Rahul Dravid can be seen nowadays advertising about High Efficiency Particle Arresting (HEPA) filters and making claims that it is important to keep the inside of your homes healthy. Indoor air quality (IAQ) is a relatively new term in Indian scenario; hence market of air filters is predicted to grow at a rapid pace. In near future it might be a common sight in Indian homes along with the now ubiquitous refrigerators, televisions and air-conditioners. As a medical student you must know about the various aspects of the purported solution being offered and the accompanying possibility of false claims.

- What is meant by indoor air quality (IAQ)?
- What are HEPA filters? Which indicators will you consider while buying one of them?
- Other than HEPA filters, name some other interventions which can improve the indoor air quality?

Guide Note

- National Biomass Cook stoves Programme (NBCP), Ministry of New and Renewable Energy.

EXERCISE 2.19

At the end of this exercise, you should be able to describe concepts of safe and wholesome water, sanitary sources of water, water purification processes, water quality standards, concepts of water conservation and rainwater harvesting **(CM3.2)**

Calculate amount of bleaching powder required to disinfect a circular well with diameter of 6 m and depth of water 12 m. The Horrock's test shows a slight blue colour in the 5th cup.

- Interpretation of above findings.

Guide Notes

- Horrock's apparatus
- Chlorination.

REFERENCES

1. Kadri's IAPSM's Textbook of Community Medicine. 2nd edn, pages 62, 69, 71, 75, 82, 86, 263, 462, 944, 967.
2. Park's Textbook of Preventive and Social Medicine. 26th edn, pages 75, 117, 175, 191, 477, 528, 799, 822, 826, 837.

FURTHER READING

1. Brain tumour risk in relation to mobile telephone use: results of the INTERPHONE international case-control study. Interphone Study Group. Int J Epidemiol. 2010 Jun; 39(3):675-94.
2. GOI Ministry of Water Resources, River development and Gang Rejuvenation. National Hydrology Project.
3. https://www.mohfw.gov.in/pdf/FinalGuidanceonMangaementofCovidcasesversion2.pdfhttps://idsp.nic.in/index1.php?lang=1andlevel=1andsublinkid=5789andlid=3722
4. Immunization Handbook for Medical Officers. New Delhi: Department of Health and Family Welfare; 2016.
5. Irish LA, Kline CE, Gunn HE, Buysse DJ, Hall MH (2015). The role of sleep hygiene in promoting public health: A review of empirical evidence. Sleep medicine reviews, 22, 23–36. https://doi.org/10.1016/j.smrv.2014.10.001.
6. Kankaria A, Nongkynrih B, Gupta SK (2014). Indoor air pollution in India: implications on health and its control. Indian journal of community medicine: official publication of Indian Association of Preventive and Social Medicine, 39(4), 203–207. https://doi.org/10.4103/0970- 0218.143019.
7. Lok Sabha unstarred question no. 1245 to be answered ON 22.12.2017 Permissible Level for Pollutants. CPCB National Ambient Air Quality Standards
8. Ministry of Law and Justice (Legislative Department) New Delhi, the 22nd April Gazette of India CG-DL-E-22042020-219108.
9. Oxford Textbook of Global Public Health 6th Edition page 1430.
10. Oxford Textbook of Public Health Page 207 volume 1
11. Page 699, 700, 750, Maxcy-Rosenau-Last – Text Book of Public Health and Preventive Medicine 15th Edition.
12. Report of the Expert Committee on Auto Fuel Policy, A technical Report by Dr R A Mashlekar https://timesofindia.indiatimes.com/india/Govt-adopts- Mashel kareport/articleshow/1691750937.cms
13. Ted Talk video on link: https://www.ted.com/talks/bill_gates_the_next_outbreak_we_re_not_ready/discussion?language=en#t-333735.
14. The Lancet (2020). India under COVID-19 lockdown. Lancet (London, England), 395(10233), 1315. https://doi.org/10.1016/S0140-6736(20)30938-7.
15. United Sates Environment Protection Agency available at https://www.epa.gov indoor-air-quality-iaq/indoor-air-quality-iaq-frequently-asked-questions.

CHAPTER

3

Epidemiology

Competency code	Competency addressed	Exercise
CM7.3	Enumerate, describe and discuss the sources of epidemiological data	3.1
CM7.4	Define, calculate and interpret morbidity and mortality indicators based on given set of data	3.1–3.4, 3.6–3.8, 3.11, 3.15–3.18, 3.20
CM7.7	Describe and demonstrate the steps in the Investigation of an epidemic of communicable disease and describe the principles of control measures	3.5
CM9.1	Define and describe the principles of demography, demographic cycle, vital statistics	3.9, 3.15
CM9.2	Define, calculate and interpret demographic indices including birth rate, death rate fertility rates	3.6, 3.8, 3.11–3.13, 3.15
CM10.1	Describe the current status of Reproductive, maternal, newborn and Child Health	3.2
CM12.1	Define and describe the concept of Geriatric services	3.7
PH1.55	Describe and discuss the following National Health programs including Immunization, Tuberculosis, Leprosy, Malaria, HIV, Filaria, Kala azar, Diarrheal diseases, Anemia and nutritional disorders, Blindness, Non-communicable diseases, Cancer and Iodine deficiency	3.10, 3.14, 3.19

EXERCISE 3.1

- At the end of this exercise, you should be able to enumerate, describe and discuss the sources of epidemiological data **(CM7.3)**
- Define, calculate and interpret morbidity and mortality indicators based on given set of data **(CM7.4)**

A village with 50,000 mid-year population, comprising of 1200 women who belong to the reproductive age group (15–49 years) for the year 2022. It was noticed that, among those 1200 women, 300 had undergone hysterectomy in the same year, due to different reasons. Bringing a total to 100, 40 new cases of women with uterine cancer in the village were identified in the year 2022.

- Mention population-at-risk in the given example
- Calculate incidence of uterine cancer in the village for year 2022.

Guide Notes

- Incidence, point and period prevalence
- Reproductive health needs.

EXERCISE 3.2

- At the end of this exercise, you should be able to define, calculate and interpret morbidity and mortality indicators based on given set of data **(CM7.4)**
- Describe the current status of reproductive, maternal, newborn and child health **(CM10.1)**

A food quality inspector report to you about an outbreak of acute gastroenteritis (AGE) originating in a restaurant. There were 15 cases of acute gastroenteritis (AGE), who ate food from that restaurant on the same day. A total of 80 people had lunch from the restaurant on that same day. As a public health specialist, you are interested in knowing morbidity profile for the same.

- Calculate attack rate of AGE
- Explain how attack rate is different from incidence rate of a disease.

Guide Notes

- Attack rate
- Incidence and prevalence
- Incubation period, window period and Latent period.

EXERCISE 3.3

At the end of this exercise, you should be able to define, calculate and interpret morbidity and mortality indicators based on given set of data **(CM7.4)**

In a society with 1500 residents, 6 people residing in the same building develop tuberculosis over a period of 5 months. Two cases were identified in January, two cases in February, one case each in April and May.

- Calculate incidence rate of tuberculosis for the month of February.
- What is the prevalence rate of tuberculosis at 5th month?
- Explain the relationship between incidence and prevalence.

Guide Note

- Point prevalence and Period prevalence.

EXERCISE 3.4

At the end of this exercise, you should be able to define, calculate and interpret morbidity and mortality indicators based on given set of data **(CM7.4)**

An outbreak of measles was reported in which 20 people in 20 different households became ill. The population of that community at that time was 1,000. One incubation period (IP) later, 10 persons among the same households of these "primary" cases developed measles. If the 20 households totaled to 80 persons, then

- What is the attack rate of measles?
- Calculate secondary attack rate of measles.

Guide Notes

- Secondary attack rate (SAR)
- Incubation period, window period and latent period.

EXERCISE 3.5

At the end of this exercise, you should be able to describe and demonstrate the steps in the investigation of an epidemic of communicable disease and describe the principles of control measures **(CM7.7)**

In a village with population of 50,000, over the years 2000–2010, a total of 15,000 incident cases of malaria were reported. During the same decade, out of 3000 total deaths reported, 100 deaths were attributed to malaria.

- What is the crude death rate for this village?
- Calculate case fatality rate due to malaria.

Guide Notes

- National Framework for Malaria Elimination
- Crude death rate
- Case fatality rate
- Other malaria-related indicators: Annual Parasite Index (API), Annual Blood Examination Rate (ABER), Slide Positivity Rate (SPR), etc.

EXERCISE 3.6

- At the end of this exercise, you should be able to define, calculate and interpret demographic indices including birth rate, death rate fertility rates **(CM9.2)**
- Enumerate, describe and discuss the sources of epidemiological data **(CM7.4)**

- At the end of this exercise, you should be able to define, calculate and interpret demographic indices including birth rate, death rate fertility rates **(CM9.2)**
- Enumerate, describe and discuss the sources of epidemiological data **(CM7.4)**

In a city with population of 1,00,000, mortality figures due to different causes, across all age groups, for the year 2015, are as follows:

Diseases	Malaria	Dengue	HTN	DM	CKD	CVA
Number of deaths	500	300	140	700	580	250

- Calculate proportional mortality from Diabetes Mellitus (DM) in the city.
- Compare proportional mortality due to communicable and non-communicable diseases and interpret the report.

Guide Notes

- Case fatality rate (CFR)
- Cause specific death rate
- Point and period prevalence
- Proportionate mortality rate.

EXERCISE 3.7

- At the end of this exercise, you should be able to define and describe the concept of Geriatric services **(CM12.1)**
- Define, calculate and interpret morbidity and mortality indicators based on given set of data **(CM7.4)**

One-year data was taken from a hospital's Medical Records Register to find mortality statistics due to diabetes mellitus. The data was segregated for different age group and is as follows:

Age group (in years)	<20	21–30	31–40	41–50	51–60	>60
Number of deaths due to DM	5	12	14	16	30	45

- Calculate proportionate mortality rate due to DM among geriatric population.

Guide Notes

- Emerging trend in NCDs
- Geriatric health needs
- Proportionate mortality rate.

EXERCISE 3.8

- At the end of this exercise, you should be able to enumerate, describe and discuss the sources of epidemiological data **(CM7.4)**
- Define, calculate and interpret demographic indices including birth rate, death rate fertility rates **(CM9.2)**

In a city with 50,000 mid-year population, a flu outbreak was reported with significant mortality in a duration of one month. Thereafter a consistent rise in the number of cases and deaths over the next four weeks was observed. A weekly data report of flu cases and associated deaths, is as below:

Week	*First*	*Second*	*Third*	*Fourth*
Cases	18	30	42	58
Deaths	3	8	16	24

- Calculate flu related weekly death rate in 3rd week of outbreak.
- Calculate death rate due to flu for the whole month.

Guide Notes

- Case fatality rate (CFR)
- Cause specific death Rate.

EXERCISE 3.9

At the end of this exercise, you should be able to define and describe the principles of demography, demographic cycle, vital statistics **(CM 9.1)**

In a city college, 500 students got admission in a year. Out of them, 350 were male students and 150 were female students.

- Calculate sex ratio for thc college for the given year.
- Calculate proportion of female students who got admission in that college in the given year.

Guide Notes

- Dependency ratio
- Sex ratio
- NFHS-5 data for India and your state.

EXERCISE 3.10

At the end of this exercise, you should be able to describe and discuss the following National Health programs including Immunization, Tuberculosis, Leprosy, Malaria, HIV, Filaria, Kala azar, Diarrheal diseases, Anemia and nutritional disorders, Blindness, Non-communicable diseases, Cancer and Iodine deficiency **(PH1.55)**

The given figure shows the occurrence of malaria at different times in a population of 500. Assuming that the population is stable at any point of time,

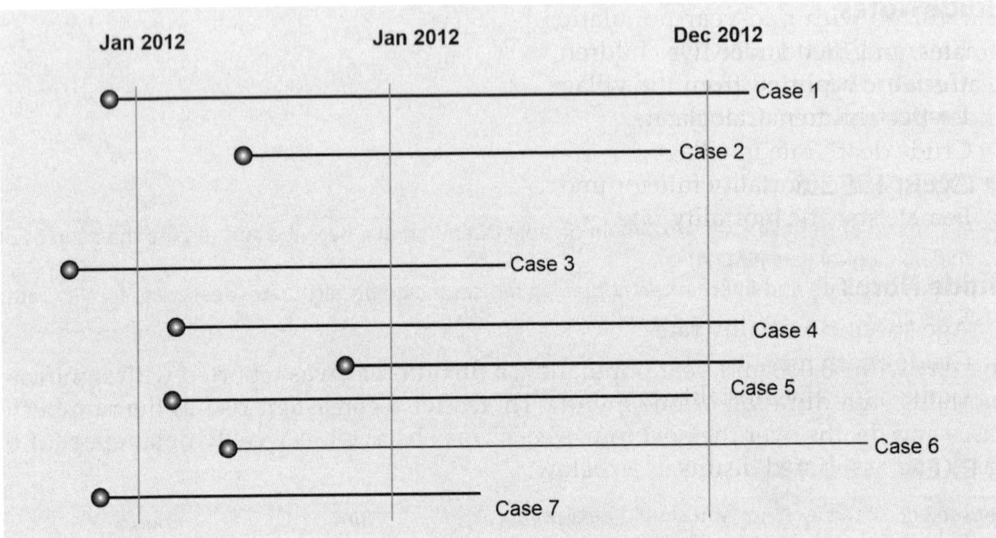

- Calculate point prevalence of malaria in January 2012
- Calculate period prevalence of malaria for the year 2012
- Calculate incidence of malaria in year 2012.

Guide Notes

- Types of incidence and prevalence
- Other malaria related indicators like ABER, API, SPR
- National Framework for Malaria Elimination.

EXERCISE 3.11

- At the end of this exercise, you should be able to enumerate, describe and discuss the sources of epidemiological data **(CM7.4)**
- Define, calculate and interpret demographic indices including birth rate, death rate fertility rates **(CM9.2)**

A health survey was conducted in a school. 100 children under the age of 5 years, were followed up for 6 months for development of any acute respiratory infections (ARI) episode. Following data has been recorded:

No. of episodes of ARI	1	2	3	4	5
No. of children	22	20	14	26	18

- Calculate measures of disease frequency among children

Guide Notes

- Measures of disease frequency
- Mortality and morbidity indicators in under-5 children.

EXERCISE 3.12

At the end of this exercise, you should be able to define, calculate and interpret demographic indices including birth rate, death rate fertility rates **(CM9.2)**

In a village with mid-year population of 20,000, there were 12,000 males and 8000 females, and 1800 under-five children, in the year 2018. For the same year, total of 300 deaths were reported from the village which includes 80 males, 130 females and 90 under-five children. Calculate:

- Crude death rate in village
- Age specific mortality rate for under-five children
- Female specific mortality rate.

Guide Notes

- Age specific mortality rate
- Crude death rate
- Gender specific mortality rate.

EXERCISE 3.13

At the end of this exercise, you should be able to define, calculate and interpret demographic indices including birth rate, death rate fertility rates **(CM9.2)**

In a city with 50,000 mid-year population, there were 200 cases of diabetes mellitus in the year 2019. Total 800 deaths occurred in the same year in the city, out of which 30 were attributable to DM. Calculate:

- Cause specific mortality rate
- Proportionate mortality ratio
- Case fatality rate.

Guide Notes

- Case fatality rate (CFR)
- Cause specific death rate
- Mortality and morbidity indicators
- Proportionate mortality rate.

EXERCISE 3.14

At the end of this exercise, you should be able to describe and discuss the following National Health programs including Immunization, Tuberculosis, Leprosy, Malaria, HIV, Filaria, Kala azar, Diarrheal diseases, Anemia and nutritional disorders, Blindness, Non-communicable diseases, Cancer and iodine deficiency **(PH1.55)**

In a Primary Health Centre with a population of 30,000 in the year 2015, malaria surveillance was conducted which revealed the following data:

- No of slides examined for malarial parasite: 1200

- No of slides positive for malaria: 30
- No of slides positive for *Plasmodium vivax*: 20
- No of slides positive for *Plasmodium falciparum*: 10

- Calculate annual blood examination rate (ABER), slide positivity rate (SPR) and annual parasite incidence (API)
- Comment on the finding of PHC survey as per guidelines of National Framework for Malaria Elimination (NFME).

Guide Notes

- ABER, API, SPR
- National Framework for Malaria Elimination.

EXERCISE 3.15

- At the end of this exercise, you should be able to enumerate, describe and discuss the sources of epidemiological data **(CM7.4)**
- Define and describe the principles of demography, demographic cycle, vital statistics **(CM9.1)**
- Define, calculate and interpret demographic indices including birth rate, death rate fertility rates **(CM9.2)**

In a village with a mid-year population of 50,000, the number of women in the reproductive age group (15–49 years) was 12000 and the number of live births in the village during that year was 3000. The mortality data of the village for the same year is as follows:

- Total deaths in village: 1500
- Early neonatal deaths: 21
- Late neonatal deaths: 9
- Deaths in children less than 1 year: 120
- Deaths in under five age group: 180
- Maternal deaths: 8

Calculate

- Maternal mortality rate and ratio
- Neonatal mortality rate
- Infant mortality rate
- Under-5 mortality rate.

Guide Notes

- ANC services utilization rate
- Infant mortality rate
- Maternal mortality rate and ratio
- Mortality and morbidity indicators in under-5 children
- Neonatal mortality rate.

EXERCISE 3.16

At the end of this exercise, you should be able to enumerate, describe and discuss the sources of epidemiological data **(CM7.4)**

In a medical oncology department, 300 patients of breast lump were screened and registered for the year 2015. Sixty cases of breast cancer were treated (surgery and chemotherapy) and followed up for a period of five years. At the end of 5 years, 10 women were reported dead.

Calculate

- 5-year survival rate for breast cancer patient in the above situation
- Case fatality rate of breast cancer.

Guide Notes

- Survival rate
- Kaplan meier curve
- Incidence, prevalence, incidence rate and density
- Interpretation of data on risk or survival
- Mortality and morbidity indicators.

EXERCISE 3.17

At the end of this exercise, you should be able to enumerate, describe and discuss the sources of epidemiological data **(CM7.4)**

An 8-year-old boy with complaints of fever and vesicular rash for 1 day came to OPD and was diagnosed with chickenpox. The same morning, he attended a class in school with a strength of 50 students. Four students in his class have had chickenpox in the past. Currently, 5 students developed similar symptoms within a period of 2 weeks.

- Calculate secondary attack rate of chickenpox
- Discuss the public health importance of SAR.

Guide Notes

- Primary case and index case
- Secondary attack rate (SAR).

EXERCISE 3.18

At the end of this exercise, you should be able to define, calculate and interpret morbidity and mortality indicators based on given set of data **(CM7.4)**

During pandemic of Influenza in 1919, basic reproduction number (R0) was reported to be 2.8. In a population of 100,000, assuming that half of the population was already immune to influenza virus, calculate:

- Effective reproduction number (R) of Influenza and interpret the results.
- What is the significance of effective reproduction number (R)?

Guide Notes

- Reproduction number (R0).

EXERCISE 3.19

At the end of this exercise, you should be able to describe and discuss the following National Health programs including Immunization, Tuberculosis, Leprosy, Malaria, HIV, Filaria, Kala Azar, Diarrheal diseases, Anemia and nutritional disorders, Blindness, Non-communicable diseases, Cancer and Iodine deficiency **(PH1.55)**

In a community with 50,000 population, a survey was conducted to search cases of lymphatic filariasis. A total of 500 persons were examined and their blood samples were collected. Only 5 out of this 500 had symptoms of lymphatic filariasis, out of which 3 had negative blood smear results.

- Calculate microfilaria rate and its endemicity rate in the given community.
- Comment on the survey's findings.

Guide Notes

- Filaria related indices
- Filariasis
- MDA for filariasis elimination.

EXERCISE 3.20

At the end of this exercise, you should be able to define, calculate and interpret morbidity and mortality indicators based on given set of data **(CM7.4)**

A village with mid-year population of 30,000 in 2020, survey was conducted to assess PHC service utilization by villagers. There were a total of 5,000 women in the reproductive age group, 30 pregnant women, out of which 21 registered their pregnancies and utilized ANC services. There were 7 maternal deaths and 2,000 live births in that year.

- Calculate maternal mortality rate and ratio
- Calculate ANC services utilization rate in village
- Comment on the findings and compare with national statistics.

Guide Notes

- ANC services utilization rate
- Maternal mortality rate and ratio
- Mortality and morbidity indicators in under-5 children.

REFERENCES

1. Kadri's IAPSM's Textbook of Community Medicine. 2nd edn, page 139.
2. Park's Textbook of Preventive and Social Medicine 25th edn, pages 65–66, 68–69, 103, 164, 287, 299, 617.
3. Park's Textbook of Preventive and Social Medicine. 26th edn, Chapter 3 'Principles of Epidemiology and Epidemiological Methods'.

FURTHER READING

1. Modern Epidemiology (3rd ed.), Rothman KJ, Lash T, Greenland S, Lippincott, Williams & Wilkins, 203.

CHAPTER 4

Research Methodology

Competency code	Competency addressed	Exercise
CM3.2	Describe concepts of safe and wholesome water, sanitary sources of water, water purification processes, water quality standards, concepts of water conservation and rainwater harvesting	4.19
CM6.1	Formulate a research question for a study	4.3, 4.6, 4.7, 4.10, 4.13, 4.14
CM6.2	Describe and discuss the principles and demonstrate the methods of collection, classification, analysis, interpretation and presentation of statistical data	4.2, 4.4, 4.13, 4.14
CM6.3	Describe, discuss and demonstrate the application of elementary statistical methods including test of significance in various study designs	4.1, 4.4, 4.14, 4.15, 4.16
CM7.1	Define epidemiology and describe and enumerate the principles, concepts and uses	4.5, 4.8, 4.11, 4.12, 4.15–4.17
CM7.3	Enumerate, describe and discuss the sources of epidemiological data	4.5, 4.6
CM7.5	Enumerate, define, describe and discuss epidemiological study designs	4.1, 4.3–4.5, 4.8–4.10, 4.12
CM7.6	Enumerate and evaluate the need of screening tests	4.1, 4.18, 4,19
CM7.8	Describe the principles of association, causation and biases in epidemiological studies	4.1, 4.2, 4.5, 4.7, 4.9, 4.10
CM14.1 CM14.2	Define and classify hospital waste Describe various methods of treatment of hospital waste	4.19 4.19

EXERCISE 4.1

- At the end of this exercise, you should be able to describe, discuss and demonstrate the application of elementary statistical methods including test of significance in various study designs **(CM6.3)**
- Enumerate, define, describe and discuss epidemiological study designs **(CM7.5)**
- Enumerate and evaluate the need of screening tests **(CM7.6)**
- Describe the principles of association, causation and biases in epidemiological studies **(CM7.8)**

In 1948, an initiative was undertaken by the US Public Health Services at Framingham, Massachusetts, USA, aimed at studying the relationship between risk factors (serum cholesterol, blood pressure, weight, and smoking) and subsequent development of cardiovascular diseases. They registered 5127 participants with multiple exposures for the study and followed them for 20 years.

- What type of study design was used?
- What is the benefit in choosing this study design?
- What did the study reveal and how did it change the disease understanding?

Guide Notes

- Types of study designs
- Steps in conducting research.

EXERCISE 4.2

- At the end of this exercise, you should be able to describe and discuss the principles and demonstrate the methods of collection, classification, analysis, interpretation and presentation of statistical data **(CM6.2)**
- Enumerate and evaluate the need of screening tests **(CM7.8)**

Comment on the following figures regarding reliability and validity.

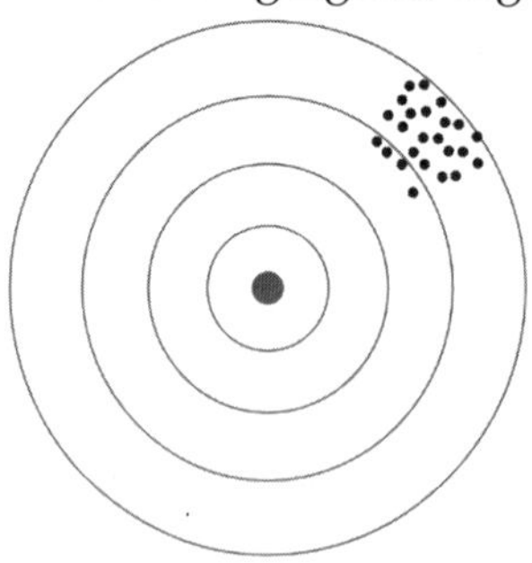

Figure: A

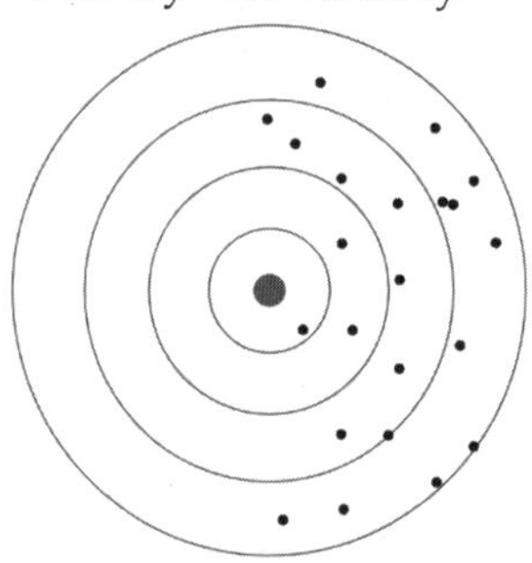

Figure: B

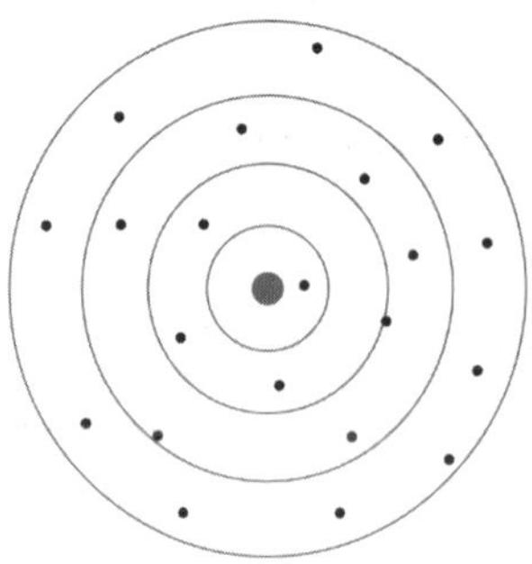

Figure: C

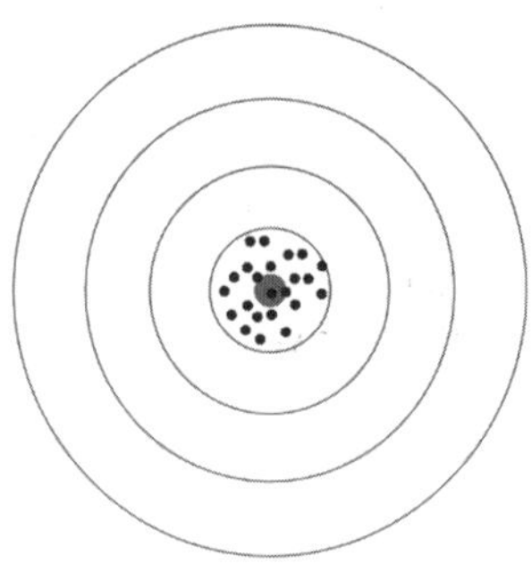

Figure: D

Guide Notes

- Consistency, precision, repeatability, reproducibility, validity of a test.
- Screening v/s diagnostic test.

EXERCISE 4.3

- At the end of this exercise, you should be able to formulate a research question for a study **(CM6.1)**
- Enumerate, define, describe and discuss epidemiological study designs. **(CM7.5)**

In 1961, a study was conducted in Federal Republic of Germany to find out the relation between thalidomide and unusual limb defects in babies born in between 1959 and 1960. They compared babies with limb defects and normal babies born in that same period. Out of 46 mothers whose gave birth to babies with typical malformations, 41 had taken thalidomide during 4th and 9th week of their pregnancies, whereas none of the 300 control mothers, whose children were normal had taken the drug at these stages.

- What type of study design was used?
- What is the benefit in choosing this study design?
- What did the study reveal and who did it changed the disease understanding?

Guide Notes

- Analytical study designs: Case control study and cohort study
- Nested case control study.

EXERCISE 4.4

- At the end of this exercise, you should be able to describe and discuss the principles and demonstrate the methods of collection, classification, analysis, interpretation and presentation of statistical data **(CM6.2)**
- Describe, discuss and demonstrate the application of elementary statistical methods including test of significance in various study designs **(CM6.3)**
- Enumerate, define, describe and discuss epidemiological study designs. **(CM7.5)**

Working as a senior researcher in a dietary research institute, you plan a study to find the relation between fatty diet and development of coronary heart disease. The data collected is represented in the following table.

	Developed coronary heart disease	***Did not develop coronary heart disease***	***Total***
Intake of high-fat diet	90	1710	1800
Intake of low-fat diet	45	1755	1800
Total	135	3465	3600

- Calculate and interpret relative risk (RR)
- Calculate Odds Ratio (OR) for this data.

Guide Notes

- Odd's ratio (OR) and Relative risk (RR)
- Categorical and continuous data
- Predictor and outcome variable.

EXERCISE 4.5

- At the end of this exercise, you should be able to define Epidemiology and describe and enumerate the principles, concepts and uses **(CM7.1)**
- Enumerate, describe and discuss the sources of epidemiological data **(CM7.3)**
- Enumerate, define, describe and discuss epidemiological study designs **(CM7.5)**
- Describe the principles of association, causation and biases in epidemiological studies **(CM7.8)**

In a study conducted by you, the incidence rate of lung cancer among smokers was found to be 10 per 1000 and among non-smokers was 1 per 1000. To what extent lung cancer can be attributed to smoking?

Guide Notes

- Attributable risk
- Confounding variable.

EXERCISE 4.6

- At the end of this exercise, you should be able to formulate a research question for a study **(CM6.1)**
- Enumerate, describe and discuss the sources of epidemiological data **(CM7.3)**

As a researcher you want to study disease and fat consumption. You plan to collect data of people affected with the disease from the hospitals and details of fat consumption from the food industry. What type of study will you choose and why?

Guide Notes

- Difference between qualitative and quantitative research
- Independent and dependent samples.

EXERCISE 4.7

- At the end of this exercise, you should be able to formulate a research question for a study **(CM6.1)**
- Describe the principles of association, causation and biases in epidemiological studies **(CM7.8)**

As a postgraduate in the surgery department, you plan your thesis where you want to do a systematic review to find out any relation between carcinoma colon and dietary fibres. During literature review you came across a study that revealed lesser incidence of carcinoma colon in pure vegetarian than non-vegetarian, by which he concluded that beta-carotene is a protective factor against cancer. This may not be true since there are many studies which reveal that high dietary fibres consumed by vegetarian subjects could also be protective against cancer. What mistake did that researcher do and how can it be rectified?

Guide Notes

- Literature review/narrative review
- Confounding variable
- Methods to remove confounding effect.

EXERCISE 4.8

- At the end of this exercise, you should be able to define epidemiology and describe and enumerate the principles, concepts and uses **(CM7.1)**
- Enumerate, define, describe and discuss epidemiological study designs. **(CM7.5)**

A study was done in 3 states to see the mean blood pressure (MBP) in each community. Health worker were assigned to visit each household in these communities. MBP in each community was calculated and compared.

- What type of study design was used?
- What are the benefits and drawbacks of this study design?

Guide Notes

- Cross-sectional study
- Objectives of descriptive and analytical research.

EXERCISE 4.9

- At the end of this exercise, you should be able to enumerate, define, describe and discuss epidemiological study designs **(CM7.5)**
- Describe the principles of association, causation and biases in epidemiological studies **(CM7.8)**

A pharmaceutical company has requested you to plan a study to test their new drug. They require that neither the patients nor the doctors should be aware of which patient is receiving the new drug and which is getting the old one. Which study type will you choose and why?

Guide Notes

- Interventional study
- Blinding in randomized control trial (RCT).

EXERCISE 4.10

- At the end of this exercise, you should be able to describe the principles of association, causation and biases in epidemiological studies **(CM7.8)**
- Formulate a research question for a study **(CM6.1)**
- Enumerate, define, describe and discuss epidemiological study designs **(CM7.5)**

You have been asked to study the effect of heavy metal consumption on the human body and the appearance of some rare diseases, for which the diagnostic tests are expensive. You have been allotted a budget and must plan a study for a longer duration. Which study type you will choose so that temporal association can be established?

Guide Notes

- Criteria for choosing analytical study
- Steps in conducting research
- Temporal association.

EXERCISE 4.11

At the end of this exercise, you should be able to define epidemiology and describe and enumerate the principles, concepts and uses **(CM7.1)**

In a population of 10000, 2000 were found to be alcoholic. Among the 10000, the people who developed cirrhosis, 70 were alcoholics and 23 were non-alcoholics. What is the population attributable risk and what do you infer from it?

Guide Notes

- Attributable risk.

EXERCISE 4.12

- At the end of this exercise, you should be able to define epidemiology and describe and enumerate the principles, concepts and uses **(CM7.1)**
- Enumerate, define, describe and discuss epidemiological study designs **(CM7.5)**

The following is the hypothetical year-wise data, regarding the sero-prevalence of Hepatitis B (per 1000) among those receiving blood transfusions from various blood banks in a city and the number of blood banks that started screening of donors for Hepatitis B prevention programme. The data was obtained from the city sero-surveillance system.

Year	***Sero-positivity in blood recipients from blood banks of city***	***Number of blood banks of the city***
2015	2.9	03
2016	2.7	04
2017	2.4	06
2018	2.1	08
2019	1.7	12
2020	1.4	16

- What conclusions can you draw from the above data?
- What kind of fallacy might be there in the above conclusion?
- What type of design is the above study?
- Is this study design a descriptive or an analytical one?

Guide Notes

- Fallacies in research.

EXERCISE 4.13

- At the end of this exercise, you should be able to formulate a research question for a study **(CM6.1)**
- Describe and discuss the principles and demonstrate the methods of collection, classification, analysis, interpretation and presentation of statistical data **(CM6.2)**

As an investigator you developed a research question as to estimate the percentage of hypertensive patients who have completely stopped salt intake as a part of prophylaxis. He defined his target population as "all hypertensive patients in the state", and the topic of interest was "the percentage of hypertensive patients who have stopped salt intake as a part of prophylaxis". He defined the study population as all patients suffering with hypertension seen at his facility during the last year and obtained the information about salt restriction by using Google form. Out of the 313 hypertensive patients who sought consultation at his facility, 290 were sent Google form link on their contact numbers (23 patients' contact number were found either invalid or incorrect). 170 patients submitted the Google form, of which a total of 61 patients reported complete cessation of salt intake. Examine the areas in this study where errors could have occurred.

Guide Notes

- Anatomy of a questionnaire
- Criteria for a good research question
- Methods of data collection.

EXERCISE 4.14

- At the end of this exercise, you should be able to formulate a research question for a study **(CM6.1)**
- Describe and discuss the principles and demonstrate the methods of collection, classification, analysis, interpretation and presentation of statistical data **(CM6.2)**
- Describe, discuss and demonstrate the application of elementary statistical methods including test of significance in various study designs **(CM6.3)**

While planning a case control study, to test the hypothesis whether a person with family history of diabetes has higher risk of developing diabetes, than the general population,

- How will you select the cases?
- How will you select controls?
- Can siblings be taken as controls, give your answer with reason?
- How will you evaluate the family history of diabetes?
- What can be the bias in this method of measurement?
- How will you measure the strength of association?
- How will you deal with the confounders?

Guide Notes

- Biases in research
- Inclusion and exclusion criteria
- Independent and dependent samples
- Steps in conducting research.

EXERCISE 4.15

- At the end of this exercise, you should be able to describe, discuss and demonstrate the application of elementary statistical methods including test of significance in various study designs **(CM6.3)**
- Define epidemiology and describe and enumerate the principles, concepts and uses **(CM 7.1)**

A new diagnostic is developed for anemia. The following table shows the finding.

Gold Std. Test ***New Test***	***Anemia Present***	***Anemia absent***
Anemia Present	300	100
Anemia Absent	25	75

- Calculate the sensitivity and specificity of this new test.

Guide Notes

- Sensitivity and specificity of a test
- Properties of tests applied in series and parallel.

EXERCISE 4.16

- At the end of this exercise, you should be able to describe, discuss and demonstrate the application of elementary statistical methods including test of significance in various study designs **(CM6.3)**
- Define Epidemiology and describe and enumerate the principles, concepts and uses **(CM7.1)**

In a population of 10000 people, the prevalence of a disease is 20%. A screening test was performed having 95% sensitivity and 80% specificity.

The positive predictive and negative predictive values of the screening test will be?

Guide Notes

- Positive predictive value (PPV) and negative predictive value (NPV) of a test.
- Properties of tests applied in series and parallel.

EXERCISE 4.17

At the end of this exercise, you should be able to define Epidemiology and describe and enumerate the principles, concepts and uses **(CM7.1)**

You are working as senior research officer at a research centre and you have been asked to comment on two newly introduced testing modalities for anemia. The following is relevant information regarding both tests.

- Test A: Sensitivity (90%) and specificity (60%)
- Test B: Sensitivity (70%) and specificity (95%)

Decide which test can be used as a screening test and which can be used as a diagnostic test.

Guide Notes

- Screening v/s diagnostic test.

EXERCISE 4.18

At the end of this exercise, you should be enumerate and evaluate the need of screening tests **(CM7.6)**

You are a private practitioner and gives consultation regarding oncological cases. A patient comes to you with her report mentioning that she has been diagnosed with carcinoma cervix. She is very worried with this report and is seeking your opinion on whether the diagnosis is correct or not and what are the chances (in percentage) that the report might be false. She had undergone a new diagnostic test which is 90% sensitive and 75% specific.

Guide Notes

- Discuss the terms: chance, risk, and odds
- Power and strength of a test.

EXERCISE 4.19

- At the end of this exercise, you should be able to describe concepts of safe and wholesome water, sanitary sources of water, water purification processes, water quality standards, concepts of water conservation and rainwater harvesting **(CM3.2)**
- Enumerate and evaluate the need of screening tests **(CM7.6)**
- Define and classify hospital waste **(CM14.1)**
- Describe various methods of treatment of hospital waste **(CM14.2)**

In your hospital's catchment area with a population of 30000, 1500 people suffered from hypothyroidism. A new diagnostic test was used, which gave true positive results in 1050 and false positive in 1900 patients. What are your comments on the new test?

Guide Notes

- Catchment area (hospital, water reservoir)
- Positive predictive value (PPV) and negative predictive value (NPV) of a test.

REFERENCES

1. Kadri's IAPSM's Textbook of Community Medicine. 2nd edn, page 167.
2. Park's Textbook of Preventive and Social Medicine. 26th edn, pages 62, 70.

CHAPTER 5

Biostatistics

Competency code	Competency addressed	Exercise
CM6.1	Formulate a research question for a particular study.	5.13
CM6.2	Describe and discuss the principles and demonstrate the methods of collection, classification, analysis, interpretation and presentation of statistical data.	5.2, 5.4, 5.11–5.13, 5.17
CM6.3	Describe, discuss and demonstrate the application of elementary statistical methods including test of significance in various study designs.	5.7–5.11, 5.16–5.18
CM6.4	Describe, discuss and demonstrate common sampling techniques, simple statistical methods, frequency distribution, measures of central tendency and dispersion.	5.1–5.6, 5.10, 5.12, 5.14, 5.19
CM7.1	Define epidemiology and describe and enumerate the principles, concepts and uses	5.6, 5.14, 5.16, 5.19
CM7.5	Enumerate, define, describe and discuss epidemiological study designs.	5.8, 5.11, 5.12, 5.15, 5.19
CM7.8	Describe the principles of association, causation and biases in epidemiological studies.	5.14
CM7.9	Describe and demonstrate the application of computers in epidemiology.	5.9
CM9.1 CM9.4	Define and describe the principles of demography, demographic cycle, vital statistics. Enumerate and describe the causes and consequences of population explosion and population dynamics of India.	5.18
PH1.55	Describe and discuss the following National Health Programme including Immunization, Tuberculosis, Leprosy, Malaria, HIV, Filaria, Kala Azar, Diarrheal diseases, Anemia and nutritional disorders, Blindness, Non- communicable diseases, cancer and Iodine deficiency.	5.13

EXERCISE 5.1

At the end of the exercise, the learner should be able to enumerate, discuss and demonstrate common sampling techniques, simple statistical methods, frequency distribution, measures of central tendency and dispersion. **(CM6.4)**

Suppose the monthly prevalence of COVID-19 patients is normally distributed with the population mean, μ = 60000, and the population standard deviation, σ =15000.

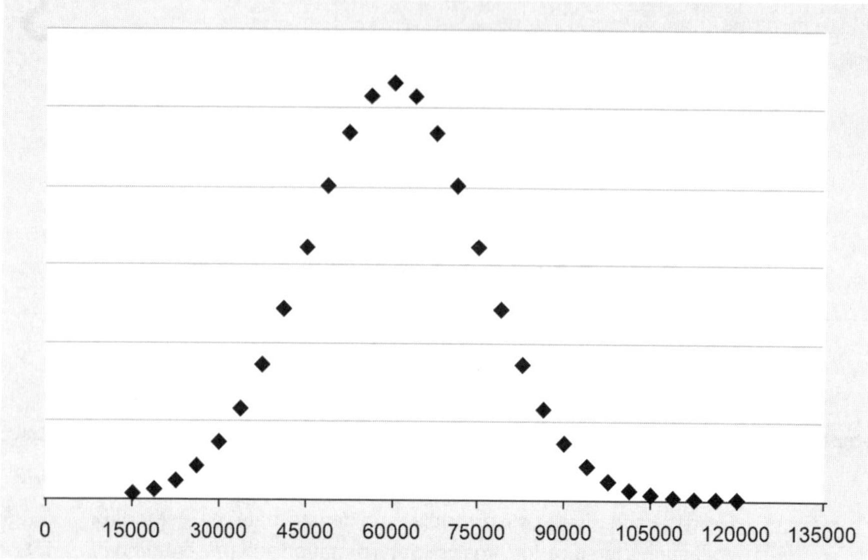

Study the above normal curve and discuss the following points:

- 16% chance of a randomly selected month having cases less than 45000
- 95% chance of a randomly selected month having cases between 30000 and 90000.

Guide Notes

- Measures of central tendency
- Measures of dispersion/variability
- Standard error, confidence interval and Z-scores.

EXERCISE 5.2

- At the end of the exercise, the learner should be able to describe and discuss the principles and demonstrate the methods of collection, classification, analysis, interpretation and presentation of statistical data. **(CM6.2)**
- Enumerate, discuss and demonstrate common sampling techniques, simple statistical methods, frequency distribution, measures of central tendency and dispersion. **(CM6.4)**

A data set showing serum iron level of 130 healthy subjects has a mean of 1.45 mg/L, median of 1.43 mg/L, mode 1.41 mg/dl and standard deviation (SD) of 0.023 mg/L.

Discuss the following points:

- The serum iron level of these healthy subjects is normally distributed, how can you justify?
- 95% of these healthy subjects have serum iron levels between 1.404 mg/L and 1.496 mg/L. Justify the statement.

Guide Notes

- Standard error, confidence Interval and Z-scores
- Types of data
- Types of distribution.

EXERCISE 5.3

At the end of the exercise, the learner should be able to describe, discuss and demonstrate common sampling techniques, simple statistical methods, frequency distribution, measures of central tendency and dispersion. **(CM6.4)**

A data set showing temperatures of a random sample of 100 frontline health providers in a COVID-19 hospital, had a mean temperature of 36.8°C and standard deviation 2.34°C.

Discuss and interpret the following findings:
- 95% Confidence interval (CI) of mean of temperature is (36.8- x 2.34, 36.8+ x 2.34)°C, considering the appropriate value of X?
- 95% of frontline health providers have temperatures between 32.12°C and 41.4 8°C
- What is the difference between the above two statements?

Guide Notes

- Measures of central tendency
- One-tailed and two-tailed distribution
- Confidence interval in one-tailed and two-tailed distribution.

EXERCISE 5.4

- At the end of the exercise, the learner should be able to describe and discuss the principles and demonstrate the methods of collection, classification, analysis, interpretation and presentation of statistical data. **(CM6.2)**
- Enumerate, discuss and demonstrate common sampling techniques, simple statistical methods, frequency distribution, measures of central tendency and dispersion. **(CM6.4)**

A data set in MS Excel of hemoglobin values (in g/dl) for 100 adolescent girls is as follows:

11.0	11.3	13.3	11.3	12.7	10.3	12.0	10.5	12.2	10.8
12.1	10.4	11.4	11.4	13.3	10.5	11.5	12.0	12.3	11.2
12.4	12.2	11.2	11.5	12.1	11.1	11.9	13.1	13.5	11.3
12.0	12.5	12.5	11.4	11.0	13.8	11.8	10.9	10.2	11.4
12.2	11.5	12.6	12.3	11.5	12.9	11.7	13.8	10.3	12.6
11.0	13.2	12.3	12.4	12.8	10.5	11.6	13.6	11.2	13.1
12.8	12.3	12.2	12.5	11.4	12.2	12.2	11.3	10.6	12.2
12.3	11.4	13.6	13.0	11.5	10.8	11.9	11.2	11.7	13.3
11.2	10.3	11.7	11.2	11.2	12.8	11.3	10.3	12.3	12.2
11.3	12.2	11.3	11.5	12.9	12.5	10.6	10.1	12.2	13.2
11.0	11.3	13.3	11.3	12.7	10.3	12.0	10.5	12.2	10.8

- Analyze the data and suggest an appropriate graph as well as comment on the distribution.
- Suggest regarding better representation of central tendency and dispersion for this data set.

Guide Notes

- Methods of data presentation
- Methods of sampling
- One-tailed and two-tailed hypothesis.

EXERCISE 5.5

At the end of the exercise, the learner should be able to enumerate, discuss and demonstrate common sampling techniques, simple statistical methods, frequency distribution, measures of central tendency and dispersion. **(CM6.4)**

Data for the heart rates (HR) of 100 healthy subjects is normally distributed and its mean is HR = 72 beats per min (bpm) with SD = 3 bpm.

- When the standard normal variate (Z) = 0.67, analyze and interpret it.
- Analyze and interpret the statement 'Area under the curve is 0.24'.

Guide Notes

- Area under the curve (AUC)
- Zone of normalcy
- Z-score.

EXERCISE 5.6

- At the end of the exercise, the learner should be able to enumerate, discuss and demonstrate common sampling techniques, simple statistical methods, frequency distribution, measures of central tendency and dispersion. **(CM6.4)**
- Define epidemiology and describe and enumerate the principles, concepts and uses. **(CM7.1)**

Suppose one study is proposed to compare the triglyceride (TG) levels between the non-vegetarian and vegetarian population. The sample size for this study was calculated to be 19 in each group, based on a previous study. [SDs are 5.7 mg/dl and 12.5 mg/dl in non-vegetarian and vegetarian groups respectively and level of significance is 0.05]. Analyze and interpret the report. To be clinically important the difference be at least 5 mg/dl in TGL levels between the two groups. Comment whether this sample size is accurate to estimate the difference? Justify your answer.

Guide Notes

- Sample size estimation
- Association, causality, correlation, and regression
- Null hypothesis (Ho) and alternate hypothesis (Ha).

EXERCISE 5.7

At the end of the exercise, the learner should be able to describe, discuss and demonstrate the application of elementary statistical methods including test of significance in various study designs. **(CM6.3)**

A study revealed that the proportion of patients of cervical cancer with five-year survival is 30%. In this case the success in this case is survival for at least 5 years [s=0.3]

$$P(x> = 7) = P(x = 7) + \ldots\ldots\ldots P(x = 10)$$
$$= 0.047$$

Analyze the above equation and interpret it.

Guide Notes

- Survival analysis/Kaplan–Meyer analysis.
- Interpretation of risk.

EXERCISE 5.8

- At the end of the exercise, the learner should be able to enumerate, define, describe and discuss epidemiological study designs **(CM7.5)**
- Describe, discuss and demonstrate the application of elementary statistical methods including test of significance in various study designs. **(CM6.3)**

A study was conducted to compare the effectiveness of the machines for use in dialysis of kidney patients. A total sample of n=70 patients with kidney disease were dialyzed by the regular machine for 1 week and 49 (70%) showed significant improvement. Next week they were dialyzed by a new machine and 56 (80%) showed significant improvement.

	Significant improvement with Machine 2		
Significant improvement with Machine 1	***Yes***	***No***	***Total***
Yes	40 (a)	09 (b)	49
No	16 (c)	05 (d)	21
Total	56	14	70

Based on this table, 95% confidence interval (CI) is (–0.04, 0.24). Analyze and interpret it.

Guide Notes

- Confidence interval (CI).

EXERCISE 5.9

- At the end of the exercise, the learner should be able to describe, discuss and demonstrate the application of elementary statistical methods including test of significance in various study designs. **(CM6.3)**
- Describe and demonstrate the application of computers in epidemiology. **(CM7.9)**

The data set of age (in years) of COVID-19 patients consists of hypothetical value of need of Hydroxychloroquine (Yes/No) by the patients, out of the total 110 patients staying in the hospital. The following data was provided. Now carry out appropriate tests to see whether HCQ is effective across the age groups or not and interpret the results.

Based on everyday experience, a practitioner asserts that 10% of total births are premature. To test this assertion, a study was conducted on a random sample of 60 births. The sample was systematically observed and 8 out of 60 births were found to be premature.

Analyze the data and comment on it.

PROPORTION STATISTICS								
		No. of premature birth	***No.***	***Proportion***	***SE of difference of proportion***	***Z-value***	***P-value***	***95% CI***
Pair 1	Study group	8	60	0.13	0.0038	0.852	0.394	(5.91% to 24.55%)
	Null hypothesis			0.10				

Guide Notes

- Hypothesis, null hypothesis (Ho) and alternate hypothesis (Ha)
- One-tailed and two-tailed hypothesis.

EXERCISE 5.13

- At the end of the exercise, the learner should be able to describe and discuss the following National Health Programme including Immunization, Tuberculosis, Leprosy, Malaria, HIV, Filaria, Kala Azar, Diarrheal diseases, Anemia and nutritional disorders, Blindness, Non- communicable diseases, cancer and Iodine deficiency. **(PH1.55)**
- Formulate a research question for a particular study. **(CM6.1)**
- Describe and discuss the principles and demonstrate the methods of collection, classification, analysis, interpretation and presentation of statistical data. **(CM6.2)**

A sample survey is planned to estimate the average level of fasting blood glucose levels in apparently healthy females aged 60 years and above, belonging to the same ethnic group. It is desired that the estimate be within 1.2 mg/dl of the population mean with a probability of 0.95. A previous study revealed an estimate of SD to be 6.3 mg/dl. The sample size for this study was found to be 106, if SRS is to be followed. If greater precision is required, what steps should be taken?

Guide Notes

- Sample size
- Simple random sampling.

EXERCISE 5.14

- At the end of the exercise, the learner should be able to enumerate, discuss and demonstrate common sampling techniques, simple statistical methods, frequency distribution, measures of central tendency and dispersion. **(CM6.4)**
- Define epidemiology and describe and enumerate the principles, concepts and uses. **(CM7.1)**
- Describe the principles of association, causation and biases in epidemiological studies. **(CM7.8)**

A prospective study was conducted to compare the risk of anemia in lower parity (<=2) with higher parity women, which had the following groups:

- Group 1–150 women with parity up to 2, and
- Group 2–150 women with higher parity The resulting table is as follows:

Women having	*Anemia*		*Total*	*Incidence*	*Relative risk*	*95%CI*	*Z-value*	*P-value*
	Yes	No						
≤2 parity	28	122	150	18.66 %	0.5833	0.3881 to 0.8767	2.593	0.009
>2 parity	48	102	150	32%				

Analyze the above observations and comment on it.

Guide Notes

- Association, covariance, and regression.

EXERCISE 5.15

At the end of the exercise, the learner should be able to enumerate, define, describe and discuss epidemiological study designs. **(CM 7.5)**

Given below is the table comparing relative risk (RR) and attributable risk (AR) of deaths due to lung cancer and COVID-19 in heavy smokers among male population residing in urban areas.

Underlying cause of death (UCoD)	*Mortality*		*RR*	*AR*
	Non-smoker	*Heavy smoker*		
Lung cancer	0.07	2.27	32.43	2.20
COVID-19	1.38	3.89	2.82	2.51

Analyze the above table and interpret it.

Guide Notes

- Relative risk (RR) and attributable risk (AR).

EXERCISE 5.16

- At the end of the exercise, the learner should be able to describe, discuss and demonstrate the application of elementary statistical methods including test of significance in various study designs. **(CM6.3)**
- Define epidemiology and describe and enumerate the principles, concepts and uses. **(CM 7.1)**

A case-control study was conducted to see the association of HIV with extramarital contacts, with the following sample sizes.

- Case- 40 promiscuous males found to be HIV
- Control- 80 (2 control: 1 case) promiscuous males of the same age and socioeconomic-cultural-ethnic background not having HIV.

The participants were asked about their sexual behavior (in terms of average frequency of extramarital contacts per year) during the last 2 years and the data obtained is as follows:

Groups	Average extramarital contacts/month		Total	Chi-square	P-value
	One or More	Less than one			
HIV+	19	21	40	5.58 df=1	
Controls	26	54	80		

Analyze the above table and interpret the findings.

Guide Notes

- Chi-square test
- Odd's ratio (OR)
- Regression models
- Statistical power of a study.

EXERCISE 5.17

- At the end of the exercise, the learner should be able to describe and discuss the principles and demonstrate the methods of collection, classification, analysis, interpretation and presentation of statistical data. **(CM6.2)**
- Describe, discuss and demonstrate the application of elementary statistical methods including test of significance in various study designs. **(CM6.3)**

A study was conducted by undergraduate students to assess the fitness and health status of the frontline health workers for COVID-19 patients. The 'VO_2 max' is taken as an indicator of fitness and health. A total of 12 participants were recruited to perform the VO_2 max test, and along with it:

- Participants' age,
- Body weight,
- Heart rate, and
- Percentage body fat were also documented.

The researcher's goal is to be able to predict VO_2 max values based on these four attributes. The data as provided in VO_2 max sheet, is shown below.

MODEL SUMMARY				
Model	R	R Square	Adjusted R Square	Std. Error of the estimate
1	0.899[a]	0.809	0.700	5.314
a. Predictors: (Constant), weight loss, % of fat, heart rate at rest, age				

ANOVA[a]						
	Model	Sum of Squares	df	Mean Square	F	Sig.
1	Regression	836.340	4	209.085	7.405	0.012[b]
Residual		197.660	7	28.237		
Total		1034.000	11			
[a]Dependent Variable: VO2 max						
[b]Predictors: (Constant), weight loss, % of fat, Heart Rate at Rest, age						

COEFFICIENTS[a]						
	Unstandardized Coefficients			***Standardized Coefficients***		
Model	***B***		***Std. Error***	***Beta***	***t***	***Sig.***
1	(Constant)	104.015	19.856		5.238	0.001
	Heart rate at rest	–0.456	0.211	–0.362	–2.161	0.068
	Percentage of fat	–0.147	0.139	–0.202	–1.059	0.325
	Age	–1.172	0.454	–0.720	–2.579	0.037
	Weight loss	–0.022	0.100	–0.058	–0.216	0.835

[a]Dependent variable: VO_{2max}

- Analyze the above tables and interpret them.
- Generate a regression equation to estimate the VO_2 max based on the four independent attributes ‘age’, ‘weight’, ‘heart rate’ and ‘percentage body fat’.

Guide Notes

- ANOVA, ANCOVA, MANCOVA
- Correlation (R) and variance (R2)
- Dependent and independent variable
- Standardization of data.

EXERCISE 5.18

- At the end of the exercise, the learner should be able to describe, discuss and demonstrate the application of elementary statistical methods including test of significance in various study designs. **(CM6.3)**
- Define and describe the principles of demography, demographic cycle, vital statistics. **(CM9.1)**
- Enumerate and describe the causes and consequences of population explosion and population dynamics of India. **(CM9.4)**

A data set of COVID-19 patients to assess the average days required for sero-conversion (positive to negative) between the patients who have taken hydroxychloroquine (HCQ) and those who have not taken the drug was obtained and is depicted in the following table:

GROUP STATISTICS							
	HCQ	***No.***	***Mean (Avg. days) of conversion***	***Std. Deviation***	***Std. Error Mean***	***T-value***	***P-value***
Negative	With medication	71	8.99	3.082	0.366	0.608 df=108	0.544
	Without medication	39	8.64	2.345	.376		

Analyze and interpret the above table.

Guide Notes

- Population parameter v/s sample statistics.
- T-value.

EXERCISE 5.19

- At the end of the exercise, the learner should be able to enumerate, discuss and demonstrate common sampling techniques, simple statistical methods, frequency distribution, measures of central tendency and dispersion. **(CM6.4)**
- Define epidemiology and describe and enumerate the principles, concepts and uses. **(CM7.1)**
- Enumerate, define, describe and discuss epidemiological study designs. **(CM7.5)**

A randomized control trial (RCT) is planned to see the difference between the efficacies of mirtazapine (new drug) and sertraline (standard drug) for the management of resistant depression over a 6-week treatment duration.

All parameters were assumed as follows: $p = 0.40$; $p0 = 0.58$; $\alpha = 0.05$; $\beta = 0.20$; $\delta = 0.18$; $\delta 0 = 0.10$. The sample size was calculated for different trials as follows:

- For Non-inferiority trial – 298
- For Equivalence trial – 378
- For statistically superiority – 121
- For Clinical Superiority – 466

Analyze and interpret the information.

Guide Notes

- Methods of sampling
- Types of trials.

REFERENCES

1. Kadri's IAPSM's Textbook of Community Medicine. 2nd edn, page 178.
2. Park's Textbook of Preventive and Social Medicine. 26th edn, page 939.

CHAPTER 6

Health Communication

Competency code	*Competency addressed*	*Exercise*
CM 1.4	Describe and discuss the natural history of disease.	6.1
CM 1.5	Describe the application of interventions at various levels of prevention.	6.1, 6.10
CM 1.6	Describe and discuss the concepts, the principles of health promotion and education, IEC and behavioral change communication (BCC).	6.1, 6.2, 6.4–6.6, 6.8–6.10
CM 1.9	Demonstrate the role of effective communication skills in health in a simulated environment	6.4–6.7
CM 1.10	Demonstrate the important aspects of the doctor patient relationship in a simulated environment	6.4, 6.5
CM 2.3	Describe and demonstrate in a simulated environment the assessment of barriers to good health and health seeking behavior.	6.10, 6.11
CM 4.1	Describe various methods of health education with their advantages and limitations	6.1, 6.4, 6.5
CM4.2	Describe the methods of organizing health promotion and education and counselling activities at individual family and community settings	6.8
CM 6.2	Describe and discuss the principles and demonstrate the methods of collection, classification, analysis, interpretation and presentation of statistical data.	6.3
IM 4.3	Discuss and describe the common causes, pathophysiology and manifestations of fever in various regions in India including bacterial, parasitic and viral causes (e.g. Dengue, Chikungunya, Typhus).	6.11
MI 8.6	Describe the basics of infection control	6.2
MI 8.7	Demonstrate infection control practices and use of personal protective equipments (PPE).	6.1, 6.2

Contd...

Competency code	*Competency addressed*	*Exercise*
CT1.18	Educate health care workers on National Program of Tuberculosis and administering and monitoring the DOTS program.	7.14
IM4.3	Discuss and describe the common causes, pathophysiology and manifestations of fever in various regions in India including bacterial, parasitic and viral causes (e.g. dengue, chikungunya, typhus).	7.1
IM9.15	Communicate the diagnosis and the treatment appropriately to patients.	7.4
IM25.1	Describe and discuss the response and the influence of host immune status, risk factors and comorbidities on zoonotic diseases (e.g. Leptospirosis, Rabies) and non-febrile infectious disease (e.g. tetanus)	7.4, 7.13
IM25.13	Counsel the patient and family on prevention of various infections due to environmental issues.	7.4
MI1.3	Describe the epidemiological basis of common infectious diseases.	7.1, 7.11
MI8.4	Describe the etiologic agents of emerging Infectious diseases.	7.13
MI8.16	Describe the National Health Programs in the prevention of common infectious disease (for information purpose only as taught in CM)	7.15
OG1.2	Define and discuss perinatal mortality and morbidity including perinatal and neonatal mortality and morbidity audit.	7.3, 7.11
OG8.1	Enumerate, describe and discuss the objectives of antenatal care, assessment of period of gestation; screening for high-risk factors.	7.4, 7.7
OG19.2	Counsel in a simulated environment, contraception and puerperal sterilisation.	7.3
OG33.3	Describe and demonstrate the screening for cervical cancer in a simulated environment.	7.12
PE3.5	Discuss the role of the child developmental unit in management of developmental delay.	7.10
PE9.1 PE9.2	Describe the age related nutritional needs of infants, children and adolescents including micronutrients and vitamins. Describe the tools and methods for assessment and classification of nutritional status of infants, children and adolescents.	7.11
PE9.7	Plan an appropriate diet in health and disease.	7.4
PE10.4	Identify children with under nutrition as per IMNCI criteria and plan referral.	7.1, 7.11
PE17.1	State the vision and outline the goals, strategies and plan of action of NHM and other important national programs pertaining to maternal and child health including RMNCH A+, RBSK, RKSK, JSSK mission Indradhanush and ICDS.	7.3, 7.4, 7.10
PE17.2	Analyze the outcomes and appraise the monitoring and evaluation of NHM.	7.3
PE18.1 PE18.2	List and explain the components, plan, and outcome of Reproductive Child Health (RCH) program and appraise its monitoring and evaluation. Explain preventive interventions for child survival and safe motherhood.	7.3, 7.4
PE18.3	Conduct antenatal examination of women independently and apply at-risk approach in antenatal care.	7.4

Contd...

Contd...

Competency code	Competency addressed	Exercise
PE18.6	Perform postnatal assessment of newborn and mother, provide advice on breast feeding, weaning and on family planning.	7.3
PE18.8	Observe the implementation of the program by visiting the Rural Health Centre.	7.1, 7.2
PE19.1	Explain the components of the Universal Immunization Program and the National Immunization Program.	7.1–7.3, 7.5, 7.15, 7.21
PE19.2	Explain the epidemiology of Vaccine preventable diseases	7.1, 7.2, 7.4, 7.5, 7.11, 7.15, 7.16
PE19.3	Vaccine description with regard to classification of vaccines, strain used, dose, route, schedule, risks, benefits and side effects, indications and contraindications.	7.1–7.5, 7.11, 7.13–7.16, 7.21
PE19.4	Define cold chain and discuss the methods of safe storage and handling of vaccines.	7.1, 7.2, 7.4–7.9, 7.11, 7.19, 7.20, 7.22
PE19.5	Discuss immunization in special situations – HIV positive children, immunodeficiency, pre-term, organ transplants, those who received blood and blood products, splenectomised children, adolescents, travelers.	7.3–7.5, 7.11, 7.12, 7.16
PE19.12	Observe the administration of UIP vaccines.	7.1, 7.2, 7.11
PE29.5	Discuss the National Anaemia Control Program.	7.4
PH1.55	Describe and discuss the following National Health Programme including immunization, tuberculosis, leprosy, malaria, HIV, filaria, kala azar, diarrheal diseases, anemiaand nutritional disorders, blindness, non-communicable diseases, cancer and Iodine deficiency.	7.11, 7.15, 7.16

EXERCISE 7.1

- At the end of the exercise, the learner should be able to Enumerate, describe and discuss the modes of transmission and measures for prevention and control of communicable and non- communicable diseases. **(CM7.2)**
- Describe and discuss the epidemiological and control measures including the use of essential laboratory tests at the primary care level for communicable diseases. **(CM8.1)**
- Enumerate and describe disease specific National Health Programs including their prevention and treatment of a case. **(CM8.3)**
- Describe and discuss the principles of planning, implementing and evaluating control measures for disease at community level bearing in mind the public health importance of the disease. **(CM8.5)**
- Describe the principles and enumerate the measures to control a disease epidemic. **(CM8.4)**
- Educate and train health workers in disease surveillance, control and treatment and health education. **(CM8.6)**
- Explain the components of the universal immunization program and the national immunization program. **(PE19.1)**
- Identify children with under nutrition as per IMNCI criteria and plan referral. **(PE10.4)**

Contd...

Contd...

- Describe various issues occurred during an outbreak and their prevention. **(CM20.2)**
- Describe the epidemiological basis of common infectious diseases. **(MI1.3)**
- Describe magnitude of problem, management, and control measures of dengue, chikungunya, typhus etc. **(IM4.3)**
- Observe the implementation of the program by visiting the Rural Health Centre. **(PE18.8)**
- Describe causative agent, host factor, environmental factor of diphtheria, tuberculosis, measles, mumps, rubella, hepatitis B, etc. **(PE19.2)**
- Discuss live/killed/both/toxoid/polysaccharide vaccine/conjugate/combined/recombinant types of vaccines, strain used, dose, route, schedule, risks, indication and contraindication of vaccines. **(PE19.3)**
- Discuss ILR, vaccine carriers, ice packs, condensation, vaccine vial monitor and Reverse cold chain. **(PE19.4)**
- Observe the step of administration of UIP vaccines. **(PE19.12)**

A case of measles was diagnosed in Hathiya village of Chaibasa, raising the concern of an outbreak. Shanti, who lives close by the case is worried that her 7-month-old daughter Pinky might contract the disease, as she has not been vaccinated against measles. She meets the local ANM and requests her to vaccinate pinky with the measles-rubella vaccine.

- What is the usual age for vaccination against measles-rubella? Which other vaccines are given along with it?
- Is it possible to modify this usual age under any specific situation(s)? Elaborate your response.
- What should the ANM do in response to Shanti's request?

Guide Notes

- National Immunization Schedule (NIS)
- Measles vaccination: vaccine, schedule, dose, route, adverse reaction, if any.
- Vaccine given along with first dose of MR/measles vaccine (2022 update).

EXERCISE 7.2

- At the end of exercise, the learner should be able to define and describe the concept of Essential Medicine List (EML). **(CM19.1)**
- Observe the implementation of the program by visiting the Rural Health Centre. **(PE18.8)**
- Explain the components of the universal immunization program and the national immunization program. **(PE19.1)**
- Describe causative agent, host factor, environmental factor of diphtheria, tuberculosis, measles, mumps, rubella, hepatitis B, etc. **(PE19.2)**
- Discuss live/killed/both/toxoid/polysaccharide vaccine/conjugate/combined/recombinant types of vaccines, strain used, dose, route, schedule, risks, indication and contraindication of vaccines. **(PE19.3)**
- Discuss ILR, vaccine carriers, ice packs, condensation, vaccine vial monitor and Reverse cold chain. **(PE19.4)**
- Observe the step of administration of UIP vaccines. **(PE19.12)**

Sapna, a newly recruited ANM is going for her first immunization session at an outreach centre in Punpun block of Patna. At the site, she needs to reconstitute the BCG vaccine but gets confused about which diluent to use. She confirms the same from another ANM via telephone and reconstitutes the BCG vaccine at 8:00 am. After administering it to 2 children, she keeps the vial in the ice pack placed on the table and continues vaccinating the children who visit her, with their age-appropriate vaccines. Just before she is about to wind up her session around 2 pm, Mini comes with her newborn twins of 5 days, requesting BCG vaccination for them.

- What is the recommended dosage of the BCG vaccine for infants?
- Describe the various diluents used for reconstitution of vaccines given under the Expanded Programme of Immunization. Which is the correct diluent to be used in the scenario described above?
- Which possible diluent can most probably be mistakenly used to reconstitute the BCG vaccine? What may happen if the said wrong diluent is used for reconstituting the BCG vaccine?
- Can the BCG vial reconstituted at 8am be used to vaccinate Mini's twins at 2 pm? Elaborate your response with the correct practice w.r.t. this case?

Guide Notes

- National Immunization Schedule (NIS)
- Correct storage and use of diluents
- BCG vaccination.

EXERCISE 7.3

- At the end of exercise, the learner should be able to define and discuss perinatal mortality and morbidity including perinatal and neonatal mortality and morbidity audit. **(OG1.2)**
- Counsel in a simulated environment, various methods of contraception and puerperal sterilization. **(OG19.2)**
- State the vision and outline the goals, strategies and plan of action of NHM and other important national programs pertaining to maternal and child health including RMNCH A+, RBSK, RKSK, JSSK mission Indradhanush and ICDS. **(PE17.1)**
- Analyze the outcomes and appraise the monitoring and evaluation of NHM. **(PE17.2)**
- List and explain the components, plan, outcome of Reproductive Child Health (RCH) program and appraise its monitoring and evaluation. **(PE18.1)**
- Explain preventive interventions for child survival and safe motherhood. **(PE18.2)**
- Perform postnatal assessment of newborn and mother, provide advice on breast feeding, weaning and on family planning. **(PE18.6)**
- Explain the components of the universal immunization program and the national immunization program. **(PE19.1)**
- Discuss live/killed/both/toxoid/polysaccharide vaccine/conjugate/combined/recombinant types of vaccines, strain used, dose, route, schedule, risks, indication and contraindication of vaccines. **(PE19.3)**
- Conduct immunization in special situations like- HIV positive children, immunodeficiency, pre-term, organ transplant, those who received blood and blood products, splenectomized children, adolescents and travelers. **(PE19.5)**
- Describe primary health care, its elements, components and principles. **(CM17.3)**

A 6-month boy Raju is brought to the CHC in Pokhran (Rajasthan) by his mother Roopa. She informed that he was born at home, delivery assisted by a local untrained *Dai* and has not received any vaccines till date.

- Which vaccines can be safely administered to Raju at this age?
- Categorize the vaccines administered to Raju as live, killed, toxoid and other preparations.
- Name the vaccines which are given in combined forms, while also mentioning its constituent antigens.

- When should Raju be given the next dose of his scheduled vaccines?
- Which vaccine(s) will not be repeated in the consequent schedule from amongst the ones administered during Raju's first visit for immunization?

Guide Notes

- National Immunization Schedule (NIS)
- Immunizing agents.

EXERCISE 7.4

- At the end of exercise the learner should be able to plan an appropriate diet in health and disease. **(PE9.7)**
- State the vision and outline the goals, strategies and plan of action of NHM and other important national programs pertaining to maternal and child health including RMNCH A+, RBSK, RKSK, JSSK mission Indradhanush and ICDS. **(PE17.1)**
- List and explain the components, plan, outcome of Reproductive Child Health (RCH) program and appraise its monitoring and evaluation. **(PE18.1)**
- Explain preventive interventions for child survival and safe motherhood. **(PE18.2)**
- Conduct antenatal examination of women independently and apply at-risk approach in antenatal care. **(PE18.3)**
- Explain the components of the universal immunization program and the national immunization program. **(PE19.1)**
- Describe causative agent, host factor, environmental factor of diphtheria, tuberculosis, measles, mumps, rubella, hepatitis B, etc. **(PE19.2)**
- Discuss live/killed/both/toxoid/polysaccharide vaccine/conjugate/combined/recombinant types of vaccines, strain used, dose, route, schedule, risks, indication and contraindication of vaccines. **(PE19.3)**
- Discuss ILR, Vaccine carriers, ice packs, condensation, vaccine vial monitor and Reverse cold chain. **(PE19.4)**
- Conduct immunization in special situations like- HIV positive children, immunodeficiency, pre-term, organ transplant, those who received blood and blood products, splenectomized children, adolescents and travelers. **(PE19.5)**
- Discuss the National Anemia Control Program. **(PE29.5)**
- Describe primary healthcare, its elements, components and principles. **(CM17.3)**
- Describe levels of healthcare delivery and its functions in India. **(CM17.5)**
- Communicate the diagnosis and the treatment appropriately to patients. **(IM9.15)**
- Describe and discuss the response and the influence of host immune status, risk factors and comorbidities on zoonotic diseases (e.g. leptospirosis, rabies) and non-febrile infectious disease (e.g. tetanus) **(IM25.1)**
- Counsel the patient and family on prevention of various infections due to environmental issues. **(IM25.13)**
- Enumerate, describe and discuss the objectives of antenatal care, assessment of period of gestation; screening for high-risk factors. **(OG8.1)**

Sadia, a 6-week pregnant woman visit the Nooranad PHC in Alappuzha (Kerala) for her ANC. After eliciting her history, careful examination and investigations, the doctor prescribes her some tablets and one injection which must be taken twice during pregnancy.

- Name the injection that may have been prescribed. What is the purpose of this injection?
- Mention the dose, route and site of administration of this injection.

- What should be the interval between two doses? In which situation, only a single dose of the said injection is recommended?
- What is the recommended storage temperature for this product and what precaution must be taken before administering the same?

Guide Notes

- National Immunization Schedule (NIS).
- Prevention of neonatal tetanus.
- Specific health protection (tetanus) under ANC.
- Vaccine safety.

EXERCISE 7.5

- At the end of exercise, the learner should be able to explain the components of the universal immunization program and the national immunization program. **(PE19.1)**
- Describe causative agent, host factor, environmental factor of diphtheria, tuberculosis, measles, mumps, rubella, hepatitis B, etc. **(PE19.2)**
- Discuss live/killed/both/toxoid/polysaccharide vaccine/conjugate/combined/recombinant types of vaccines, strain used, dose, route, schedule, risks, indication and contraindication of vaccines. **(PE19.3)**
- Discuss ILR, Vaccine carriers, ice packs, condensation, vaccine vial monitor and Reverse cold chain. **(PE19.4)**

The vaccination of one 7-month Zinia had been discontinued after an episode of persistent inconsolable screaming (>3 hours) following immunization at 6 weeks. After weeks of counselling by the Anganwadi worker (AWW) and the neighbour, her mother again brought her to the AWC at this age to get the remaining vaccines administered.

- Name the vaccine and its component that may have been responsible for the persistent screaming episode following immunization at 6 weeks.
- What can be done to avoid this kind of untoward reaction in the subsequent vaccination schedules?
- Should the vaccination schedule be restarted all over again? Elaborate your answer.

Guide Notes

- *DPT vaccine:* Preparation, schedule, dose, route, placement in the cold chain, AEFI and contraindications.
- *All other vaccines:* Preparation, schedule, dose, route, placement in the cold chain, AEFI and contraindications.

EXERCISE 7.6

- At the end of the exercise, the learner should able to discuss ILR, vaccine carriers, ice packs, condensation, vaccine vial monitor and Reverse cold chain. **(PE 19.4)**

On a chilly winter morning in Leh, Wangmo Dolma, the ANM, reaches the Spituk PHC to begin her day's work. As she opens the ILR to fetch the vaccines for sending them off to the session sites, she realizes that the thermometer is showing sub-zero temperature. She panics for a moment and hurriedly takes out some specific vaccine vials and thoroughly inspects them. She does not notice anything unusual, but her concerns remain unaddressed.

- What do you think Wangmo Dolma is so concerned about?
- Enlist the vaccines that may be related to her concern.
- What was she expecting to see while inspecting the vaccine vials?
- What should she do to be satisfied that her concerns are addressed? Explain the steps in correct order.

Guide Note

- Cold chain (sensitivity to heat and freezing and freeze damage to the vaccine).

EXERCISE 7.7

- At the end of exercise, the learner should be able to enumerate, describe and discuss the objectives of antenatal care, assessment of period of gestation; screening for high-risk factors. **(OG8.1)**
- Discuss ILR, vaccine carriers, ice packs, condensation, vaccine vial monitor and reverse cold chain. **(PE19.4)**

Sarita is a graduate and works as an assistant in a private firm in Noida. She had a complicated pregnancy, and her first child Ankit was born when she was 37 years old. When she took him to the Bhangel PHC in Noida for his vaccination, due at 6 weeks, she was horrified to see that the ANM was vaccinating her child from a previously opened vial. She raised a hue andcry about the same and insisted that a new vial be opened to vaccinate Ankit.

- Is it acceptable to use vials opened in previous sessions to immunize infants? What is this practice/policy called?
- Which vaccines can be used in this manner?
- What are the conditions that need to be fulfilled for this practice?

Guide Note

- Open vial policy.

EXERCISE 7.8

At the end of the exercise, the learner should able to discuss ILR, vaccine carriers, ice packs, condensation, vaccine vial monitor and reverse cold chain. **(PE 19.4)**

During the monitoring activities of the pulse polio campaign in Manihari block of Katihar (Bihar), the external monitor Dr Suhas spotted two ladies in yellow sleeveless jackets near a tea stall. It was a sunny day, and they were sitting in the open nonchalantly chatting with each other while the vaccine carrier was also kept on the pavement next to them. He identified them as polio workers, approached them and introduced himself as a monitor.To his obvious question of what they were doing there instead of vaccinating children, they replied that they had finished their task just a few moments ago and were now waiting for a vehicle to go to the PHC for the evening meeting. Dr Suhas examined the tally sheets, inspected the vaccine vial labels, asked them some questions, and left after giving them some friendly professional advice.

- What is the pulse polio campaign?
- Was it correct to keep the vaccine carrier directly under the sun? If not, why?
- What are the important things that Dr Suhas may have checked on the vaccine vial labels? What is the significance of checking the same? Describe how this may be interpreted.

Guide Notes

- Pulse polio campaign
- Vaccine vial monitor.

EXERCISE 7.9

- At the end of the exercise, the learner should able to discuss ILR, Vaccine carriers, ice packs, condensation, vaccine vial monitor and reverse cold chain. **(PE 19.4)**

On resuming her duty, after maternity leave, at the PHC, Churaut in Sitamarhi (Bihar), ANM Anita Devi was aghast to see the condition of the ILR. All the vaccines were stocked in a haphazard manner. The other ANM Roksana, who was working as her substitute, when asked, responded that she was not sure about how exactly the vaccines were meant to be stored in the ILR. Anita also observed that Roksana had taken out the ice packs from the deep freezer (DF) and directly placed them in the vaccine carriers to be sent for outreach sessions.

- Is there any specified order of storing vaccines in the ILR? Why do you think so?
- What is the correct order of storing vaccines in the ILR?
- What is the significance of Anita's observation of the ice packs being placed into the vaccine carriers immediately after being taken out of the DF?
- What is the ideal practice for using ice packs? What is the name of this practice?

Guide Notes

- Temperature requirements for vaccines
- Electrical cold chain equipment (ILR)
- Conditioning of ice packs.

EXERCISE 7.10

- At the end of exercise, the learner should be able to state the vision and outline the goals, strategies and plan of action of NHM and other important national programs pertaining to maternal and child health including RMNCH A+, RBSK, RKSK, JSSK mission Indradhanush and ICDS. **(PE 17.1)**
- Discuss the role and responsibilities of the child developmental unit in management of developmental delay. **(PE 3.5)**

While planning the activities of Mission Indradhanush, Sadia, the ANM, informed the MOIC of Maner PHC, Dr. Ramjivan Singh that she had recently spotted a small settlement of labourers and their families near the new brick kilns that have come up in the Haldi Chhapra area. There were some young children and infants among them. Sadia also overheard while crossing the grapevines that a group of transgenders living in Maner had recently brought with them a newborn with unambiguous genitalia, whom they found abandoned near the village temple. They are now going to raise the child as one of them.

- What is Mission Indradhanush? When was it launched in India?
- What will be the modus operandi to ensure coverage of infants/children and/or pregnant women living in these temporary settlements around the brick kilns in this area?
- What is the significance of the information regarding the adoption of the baby with unambiguous genitalia by a group of transgender?

Guide Notes

- Mission Indradhanush
- Intensified Mission Indradhanush (IMI)
- *Confuser:* Abhiyan Indradhanush

EXERCISE 7.11

- At the end the this exercise the learner should be able to describe the age related nutritional needs of infants, children and adolescents including micronutrients and vitamins. **(PE9.1)**
- Describe the tools and methods for assessment and classification of nutritional status of infants, children and adolescents. **(PE9.2)**
- Describe causative agent, host factor, environmental factor of Diphtheria, tuberculosis, measles, mumps, rubella, hepatitis B, etc. **(PE19.2)**
- Discuss live/killed/both/toxoid/polysaccharide vaccine/conjugate/combined/recombinant types of vaccines, strain used, dose, route, schedule, risks, indication and contraindication of vaccines. **(PE19.3)**
- Discuss ILR, vaccine carriers, ice packs, condensation, vaccine vial monitor and Reverse cold chain. **(PE19.4)**
- Describe and discuss the epidemiological and control measures including the use of essential laboratory tests at the primary care level for communicable diseases. **(CM8.1)**
- Describe the epidemiological basis of common infectious diseases. **(MI1.3)**
- Discuss aims, objectives, strategy, milestones, treatment, and preventive part of respective national programme. **(PH1.55)**
- Describe Universal Immunization Program; Integrated Management of Neonatal and Childhood Illness (IMNCI) and other existing programs. **(CM10.5)**
- Identify children with under nutrition as per IMNCI criteria and plan referral. **(PE10.4)**
- Define and discuss perinatal mortality and morbidity including perinatal and neonatal mortality and morbidity audit. **(OG1.2)**

Somshukla, who works as a domestic help in a household in Howrah (West Bengal), has a 3-month- old daughter, who has been having multiple episodes of diarrhea since last night. Recently, one of her neighboring family had lost their infant due to diarrhea. She is apprehensive about a similar outcome, as she has been careless to the extent of not even continuing her daughter's immunization after the birth doses. Hence, she decides to take her to a nearby health facility. However, before that, she visits her employers to request a day's leave and some advance. On hearing her plight, Mrs. Bose, her employer, gave her some money and a day's leave. She also told Somshukla to keep giving fluids to the baby and mentions a vaccine that she recently heard about; one that protects children from diarrhea.

- Name the vaccine that Mrs Bose might have mentioned about. Will immunization with this vaccine prevent all kinds of diarrhea?
- What is the maximum age till which the first dose of this vaccine can be given? Is a booster dose required?
- Is the open vial policy applicable to this vaccine? Elaborate.

Guide Notes

- Rotavirus vaccine
- Causes of diarrhea.

EXERCISE 7.12

- At the end of the exercise, the learner should be able to conduct immunization in special situations like- HIV positive children, immunodeficiency, pre-term, organ transplant, those who received blood and blood products, splenectomized children, adolescents and travelers. **(PE19.5)**
- Describe the physiology, clinical management and principles of adolescent health including ARSH. **(CM10.8)**
- Describe and demonstrate the screening for cervical cancer in a simulated environment. **(OG33.3)**

The department of Women's Studies in Delhi University had organized a workshop on adolescent health recently. Rina, who works as a lecturer in the department, was made the coordinator for this workshop. During one of the sessions, while she was passing through the corridor, the mention of cervical cancer caught her attention, as her mother was recently diagnosed with the same. So, she went inside the hall and started listening intently. Thinking of her ailing mother and her suffering, she was filled with sadness and despair until the expert speaker, Dr Neha started deliberating on the preventive components of screening for and vaccination against the disease. She was elated at the thought that her young daughter of 11 years would not have to suffer the same fate as her mother, if she received the vaccine to prevent the cancer, so she decided to take her daughter to a renowned gynecologist to get the vaccine the very next day.

- Which vaccine can prevent cervical cancer? What are the two main varieties of this vaccine which are commonly available for vaccination?
- What other conditions can be prevented by the vaccine type that includes more strains of the HPV?
- How many doses of this vaccine should be given to Rina's daughter at this age? Is there any difference in the number of doses for different age groups?
- What is the ideal time for vaccination against HPV?

Guide Notes

- HPV vaccination recommended for all healthy adults
- Prevention and control of cancer cervix
- Indigenous HPV vaccine developed in India (in 2022).

EXERCISE 7.13

- At the end of this exercise the learner should be able to describe the etiologic agents, course and diagnosis of emerging infectious diseases. **(MI8.4)**
- Describe and discuss the response and the influence of host immune status, risk factors and comorbidities on zoonotic diseases (e.g. leptospirosis, rabies) and non-febrile infectious disease (e.g. tetanus) **(IM25.1)**
- Discuss live/killed/both/toxoid/polysaccharide vaccine/conjugate/combined/recombinant types of vaccines, strain used, dose, route, schedule, risks, indication and contraindication of vaccines. **(PE19.3)**

Like every day at dawn, Mahesh, a newspaper vendor, was riding his bicycle on his way to collect newspapers for distribution. Just as he was about to reach the depot, he saw a group of 6–7 dogs fighting amongst themselves on the street. Without giving much thought, he continued to move ahead but unfortunately something flew in his eye, he lost his balance and fell. The dogs were very close to where Mahesh fell and pounced over him. He started shrieking in fear and pain as they scratched and bit him at multiple spots. He was taken to the nearest health facility by other vendors present at the depot, who also rescued him from the attack. The doctor on examination found his bite injuries to be of category III. He advised thorough washing of the wounds with soap and running water, administered three kinds of injections, including one dose of Tetvac injection and asked him to return for subsequent doses of the vaccine.

- What are the other two kinds of injections that were prescribed along with Tetvac injection?
- How do they confer protection from bite complications?
- Describe the post exposure prophylaxis (PEP) in such situations.
- What is the latest method of inducing passive immunity after a dog bite?

Guide Notes

- National rabies control program
- Post exposure prophylaxis of rabies
- Rabies human monoclonal antibodies.

EXERCISE 7.14

- At the end of the exercise, the learner should able to discuss live/killed/both/toxoid/polysaccharide vaccine/conjugate/combined/recombinant types of vaccines, strain used, dose, route, schedule, risks, indication and contraindication of vaccines. **(PE19.3)**
- Describe and discuss the epidemiology of tuberculosis and its impact on the work, life and economy of India. **(CT1.1)**
- Prescribe an appropriate anti-tuberculosis regimen based on the location of disease, smear positivity and negativity and co- morbidities based on current national guidelines including directly observed tuberculosis therapy (DOTS). **(CT1.15)**
- Describe the appropriate precautions, screening, testing and indications for chemoprophylaxis for contacts and exposed health care workers. **(CT1.16)**
- Educate healthcare workers on National Program of Tuberculosis and administering and monitoring the DOTS program. **(CT1.18)**

Like usual days, Dr Koteswara Rao went to the PHC in Bibinagar (Telangana), where he was posted as a Medical Officer. Owing to the 3 deliveries he took a night before; he was feeling fatigued because of insufficient sleep. On the present-day duty, he was faced with a worried mother Parimala, who had created ruckus about development of an ulcer on the left arm of his newborn son, Ashwin, a few weeks after his first immunization at birth. Despite all efforts by the ANM and other staff members to calm her down, she did not listen and hence Dr Rao finally intervened and assured her that it was an expected outcome and that there was no risk to the health or life of the child. It was only after this constant assurance that she was finally convinced and went home.

- Which vaccine is given in the left upper arm at birth? Mention its full name and the strain used to manufacture the vaccine.
- Why are vaccines always given at a specified spot in the body?
- What did Dr Rao mean when he said it was an "expected outcome"? Describe.
- Is it necessary to repeat the dose of the vaccine if no scar has developed as sequelae of vaccination?

Guide Note

- BCG vaccination

EXERCISE 7.15

- At the end of exercise, the learner should be able to describe the National Health Programs in the prevention of common infectious disease (for information purpose only as taught in CM) **(MI8.16)**
- Discuss aims, objectives, strategy, milestones, treatment, and preventive part of respective National programme. **(PH1.55)**
- Explain the components of the universal immunization program and the national immunization program. **(PE19.1)**
- Describe causative agent, host factor, environmental factor of Diphtheria, tuberculosis, measles, mumps, rubella, hepatitis B, etc. **(PE19.2)**
- Discuss live/killed/both/toxoid/polysaccharide vaccine/conjugate/combined/recombinant types of vaccines, strain used, dose, route, schedule, risks, indication and contraindication of vaccines. **(PE19.3)**

At a session site, somewhere in the remote areas of Chitrakoot (MP), Sultana, an ANM was passing some key messages to the mothers of children who were immunized therein. During this exercise, she happened to mention an injection against polio, which startled Gauri, who had brought her 6-week-old daughter Nima for immunization. Gauri lived in the city before being married into the village and was 12th pass. She considered herself better aware than most other women in the village. As awareness about the oral administration of polio vaccine is a common place, she raised an objection on the need for an injectable polio vaccine.

- What 4 key messages the ANM might have given to the mothers of children at the session site?
- What is IPV? Can OPV be given in place of IPV?
- Is it safe to give the oral and injectable Polio vaccines together?

Guide Notes

- Inactivated polio vaccine (IPV) in NIS
- Managing an immunization session, with emphasis on communicating with each beneficiary
- 2022 guideline for the 3rd dose of fIPV.

EXERCISE 7.16

- At the end of the exercise, the learner should able to describe causative agent, host factor, environmental factor of diphtheria, tuberculosis, measles, mumps, rubella, hepatitis B, etc. **(PE19.2)**
- Discuss live/killed/both/toxoid/polysaccharide vaccine/conjugate/combined/recombinant types of vaccines, strain used, dose, route, schedule, risks, indication and contraindication of vaccines. **(PE19.3)**
- Conduct immunization in special situations like-HIV positive children, immunodeficiency, pre-term, organ transplant, those who received blood and blood products, splenectomized children, adolescents and travelers. **(PE19.5)**
- Discuss aims, objectives, strategy, milestones, treatment, and preventive part of respective national programme. **(PH1.55)**
- Describe various issues occurred during an outbreak and their prevention. **(CM20.2)**

During the preparatory exercises preceding the Measles Rubella Vaccination Campaign (MRVC) in Bhopal, the District Immunization Officer (DIO), Dr Safdar Khan went with a team of health workers to a local *madrassa*, which had communicated its reluctance in allowing its students to be vaccinated after the *maulvi* had received some disturbing videos on WhatsApp about targeting a certain community in the name of MRVC by injecting them with drugs that will affect their fertility and growth. It took Dr. Khan, a great deal of convincing, before the maulvi finally agreed to participate and support the campaign.

- What is the measles rubella vaccination campaign?
- What is the phenomenon of such reluctance towards vaccination called? Explain.
- Mention the determinants of this phenomenon.

Guide Notes

- Measles rubella vaccination campaign
- Vaccine hesitancy.

EXERCISE 7.17

At the end of this exercise the learner should be able to educate and train health workers in disease surveillance, control & treatment and health education. **(CM8.6)**

During the review meeting of state AEFI committee of Punjab, a cluster of four cases developing sterile abscess was reported from an Anganwadi Centre (AWC) in Gurdaspur following immunization with the pentavalent vaccine. Further description of the situation revealed that the ANM, Gurpreet, appointed there was not trained on immunization and was substituting for her sister who was not well that day. She had observed precipitate inside the vaccine vial but was oblivious to the significance of the same. Hence, she administered the vaccine without giving it much thought.

- What is an event of this nature called? Define and mention its significance.
- How are these events categorized? Mention the category of the event described in the above case study.
- What can be done to prevent such events?

Guide Notes

- AEFI and its management at community level
- Clustering of AEFI.

EXERCISE 7.18

- At the end of the exercise, the learner should able to discuss ILR, Vaccine carriers, ice packs, condensation, vaccine vial monitor and reverse cold chain. **(PE19.4)**
- Describe and demonstrate the application of computers in epidemiology. **(CM7.9)**

As part of the EVM assessment in Assam, a team comprising of Dr Sinha and Dr Saikiya visited the Harangajao PHC in Dima Hasao district. They were satisfied to see that eVIN was installed with the ILR. However, the cold chain handler Vaiphei was only using it as a temperature monitoring device because she had not been trained to use it effectively. The team also observed that the generator was not in working order reportedly from the last 2 days and this had been intimated to the District Immunization Office for sending a technician to repair the same. Hence in the event of a power failure or equipment breakdown they were using the contingency plan which was clearly displayed on a poster in the cold chain room. The team carefully noted these observations for mentioning in their report submitted to the state for necessary support and improvement in the long run.

- What is EVM assessment? What role does it play in the immunization programme?
- What is eVIN?
- What do you understand by contingency plan?

Guide Notes

- Global EVM initiative
- Cold chain management.

EXERCISE 7.19

- At the end of the exercise, the learner should able to discuss ILR, Vaccine carriers, ice packs, condensation, vaccine vial monitor and Reverse cold chain. **(PE19.4)**

As the time for the launch of the Rotavirus vaccine in her state came closer, Urvi, a pharmacist, who had been assigned the additional responsibility of handling the cold chain at the Gaul PHC in Wardha district, started preparing for the smooth rollout of the vaccine introduction in her block. She started with the estimation of vaccine requirement to send the demand to the district vaccine store. Since vaccines are usually received by the pull mechanism and this was the first lot of vaccines that the PHC would receive, she wanted to ensure that the buffer stock remained adequate should there be any delay in the subsequent vaccine supply due to prolonged lead time or unforeseen wastage of the vaccine.

- How will Urvi calculate the rotavirus vaccine requirement for her block?
- What do you understand by the pull and push mechanism?
- Define buffer stock and lead time.
- What is the method of estimating the wastage rate of vaccines? What are the reasons for wastage of unopened vials?

Guide Notes

- Estimation of vaccine requirements
- Wastage rate
- Planning for vaccination at health centers.

EXERCISE 7.20

At the end of the exercise, the learner should able to discuss ILR, vaccine carriers, ice packs, condensation, vaccine vial monitor and reverse cold chain. **(PE19.4)**

As part of his monthly monitoring activities, the district immunization officer of Doda, Dr Nasir visited the Humbal PHC. He observed that there was a small ILR in which all the vaccines were kept, and it seemed a little overcrowded. The good thing was that all the vaccines were arranged meticulously in the correct order. However, on further exploration he figured that while arranging the vaccine the consideration of EEFO and FIFO had not been given due importance. Since he was aware about the plan of introduction of the rotavirus vaccine (RVV) in the next two months, and anticipated that a larger ILR will be needed to accommodate all the vaccines in the future. The DIO gave some onsite training to the cold chain handler, Sunny, to further arrange the vaccines based on EEFO and FIFO principles and instructed him to send requisition for a larger ILR keeping in mind the requirement of additional storage space in the coming months.

- What do you understand by EEFO and FIFO? When can an exception be made to the same?
- Considering the impending introduction of RVV in the coming months, how will the cold chain handler calculate the net storage volume for the vaccine to be stored in the ILR?

Guide Notes

- Assessing the cold chains space and inventory
- Planning for vaccines and drugs at health centers.

EXERCISE 7.21

- At the end of exercise, the learner should be able to explain the components of the universal immunization program and the national immunization program. **(PE19.1)**
- Discuss live/killed/both/toxoid/polysaccharide vaccine/conjugate/combined/recombinant types of vaccines, strain used, dose, route, schedule, risks, indication and contraindication of vaccines. **(PE19.3)**

Lopamudra is posted as an ANM at a sub-centre of PHC Jharapada in Bhubaneshwar, which caters to a population of 4800, out of which the number of pregnant women is 220. She needs to carry out immunization session for women who come for their ANC visits and has to develop a micro plan in accordance with that.

- What is the schedule for TT vaccine during pregnancy?
- What is the requirement of TT vaccine vial per month?
- What is the requirement of syringes per month?

Guide Notes

- National Immunization Schedule (NIS)
- Planning Immunization Services.

EXERCISE 7.22

- At the end of the exercise, the learner should able to discuss ILR, Vaccine carriers, ice packs, condensation, vaccine vial monitor and Reverse cold chain. **(PE19.4)**

In a PHC covering population of 40,000 with CBR of 20/1000 mid-year population and IMR of 40/1000 live-births.

- Calculate vaccine requirement for one year time.

Guide Note

- Calculation of vaccine requirement and vaccine wastage.

REFERENCES

1. Kadri's IAPSM's textbook of Community Medicine. 2nd ed, pages 231, 255, 364, 459, 821, 892, 965, 967, 973, 974.
2. Park's Textbook of Preventive and Social Medicine. 26th ed, pages 117, 120-121, 135, 258, 317, 355, 434, 497.

FURTHER READING

1. Immunization Handbook for Health Workers 2018.
2. Measles Rubella Vaccine Operational Guidelines.
3. National EVM assessment handbook 2018 (https://www.nhm.gov.in/New_Updates_2018/NHM_Components/Immunization/Guildelines_for_ immunization/National_EVM_Assessment_Report_2018.pdf).
4. Operational guidelines for introduction of Rotavirus vaccine in the UIP.
5. Report of the sage working group on vaccine hesitancy (https://www.who.int/immunization/sage/meetings/2014/october/SAGE_working_group_revised_ report_vaccine_hesitancy.pdf?ua=1).

CHAPTER

8

Infectious Diseases

Competency code	Competency addressed	Exercise
CM1.5	Describe the application of interventions at various levels of prevention	8.4
CM3.3	Describe the aetiology and basis of water borne diseases/jaundice/ hepatitis/diarrheal diseases	8.7, 8.8, 8.10, 8.17
CM5.3	Define and describe common nutrition related health disorders (including macro-PEM, Micro-iron, Zn, iodine, Vit. A), their control and management	8.7, 8.18
CM7.7	Describe and demonstrate the steps in the investigation of an epidemic of communicable disease and describe the principles of control measures	8.1
CM8.1	Describe and discuss the epidemiological and control measures including the use of essential laboratory tests at the primary care level for communicable diseases	8.1, 8.2, 8.12–8.15
CM8.3	Enumerate and describe disease specific National Health Programs including their prevention and treatment of a case.	8.2, 8.12, 8.15
CM8.5	Describe and discuss the principles of planning, implementing and evaluating control measures for disease at community level bearing in mind the public health importance of the disease.	8.1, 8.2, 8.11–8.15
CM10.5	Describe Universal Immunization Program; Integrated Management of Neonatal and Childhood Illness (IMNCI) and other existing programs	8.7, 8.14, 8.16–8.18
CM20.2	Describe various issues occurred during an outbreak and their prevention	8.1
IM4.3	Discuss and describe the common causes, pathophysiology and manifestations of fever in various regions in India including bacterial, parasitic and viral causes (e.g. dengue, chikungunya, typhus)	8.5
MI1.3	Describe the epidemiological basis of common infectious diseases.	8.1, 8.5, 8.6, 8.8–8.10, 8.15
MI8.4	Describe the etiologic agents, course and diagnosis of emerging infectious diseases	8.1
PE3.5	Discuss the role of the child developmental unit in management of developmental delay.	8.2
PE3.7	Visit a child developmental unit and observe its functioning.	8.2
PE8.1	Define the term complementary feeding.	8.16
PE8.2	Discuss the principles, the initiation, attributes, frequency, techniques and hygiene related to complementary feeding including IYCF.	8.2, 8.16

Contd...

Contd...

Competency code	*Competency addressed*	*Exercise*
PE8.3	Enumerate the common complementary foods.	8.16
PE8.4	Elicit history on the complementary feeding habits.	8.2, 8.16
PE8.5	Counsel and educate mothers on the best practices in complementary feeding.	8.2, 8.16
PE9.1	Describe the age related nutritional needs of infants, children and adolescents including micronutrients and vitamins.	8.2, 8.14, 8.16
PE9.2	Describe the tools and methods for assessment and classification of nutritional status of infants, children and adolescents.	8.2, 8.14, 8.16
PE9.5	Calculate the age related calorie requirement in health and disease and identify gap.	8.2, 8.16
PE9.6	Assess and classify the nutrition status of infants, children and adolescents and recognize deviations.	8.2, 8.16
PE10.4	Identify children with under nutrition as per IMNCI criteria and plan referral.	8.2, 8.7, 8.14, 8.16
PE17.1	State the vision and outline the goals, strategies and plan of action of NHM and other important national programs pertaining to maternal and child health including RMNCH A+, RBSK, RKSK, JSSK mission Indradhanush and ICDS.	8.2, 8.17
PE19.1 PE19.2 PE19.3	Explain the components of the universal immunization program and the national immunization program. Explain the epidemiology of vaccine preventable diseases Vaccine description with regard to classification of vaccines, strain used, dose, route, schedule, risks, benefits and side effects, indications and contraindications.	8.2–8.4, 8.6
PE19.4	Define cold chain and discuss the methods of safe storage and handling of vaccines.	8.3, 8.4
PE19.5	Discuss immunization in special situations- HIV positive children, immuno-deficiency, pre-term, organ transplants, those who received blood and blood products, splenectomised children, adolescents, travelers.	8.9
PH1.55	Describe and discuss the following National Health Programmes including immunization, tuberculosis, leprosy, malaria, HIV, filaria, kala azar, diarrheal diseases, anemia and nutritional disorders, blindness, non-communicable diseases, cancer and iodine deficiency	8.7, 8.17

EXERCISE 8.1

- At the end of this exercise, the learner should able to describe and demonstrate the steps in the investigation of an epidemic of communicable disease and describe the principles of control measures. **(CM7.7)**
- Describe and discuss the epidemiological and control measures including the use of essential laboratory tests at the primary care level for communicable diseases. **(CM8.1)**
- Describe the etiologic agents, course and diagnosis of emerging Infectious diseases. **(MI8.4)**
- Describe and discuss the principles of planning, implementing and evaluating control measures for disease at community level bearing in mind the public health importance of the disease. **(CM8.5)**
- Describe various issues occurred during an outbreak and their prevention. **(CM20.2)**
- Describe the epidemiological basis of common infectious diseases. **(MI1.3)**

In a tertiary care teaching institute, a nursing student reported to the OPD with a history of fever for 2 days, followed by lesions on face, chest, and back, which later spread to the whole body. The lesions were vesicular in nature. She was unaware of any contact with a chicken pox infected case at home or in the hospital. Upon consultation with her supervisor, it was found that she was posted in the Pulmonary ICU, where a case of rashes was treated nearly 2 weeks ago. Her vaccination history revealed that she was neither vaccinated nor had an infection of varicella before. Two days later, a resident doctor and two nurses reported with similar history and clinical manifestation and were also found to be posted in Pulmonary ICU. Five nurses and two residents from that ICU reported with fever and vesicular lesions within one week of the first case. All the nurses and residents were started on treatment and were asked to isolate themselves. The investigation of epidemic was started after the matter was reported to infection control committee.

- What is the probable diagnosis?
- What are the complications of this disease?
- What are the next steps in management of the disease outbreak?

Guide Notes

- Epidemiology of chickenpox
- Steps of outbreak investigation.

EXERCISE 8.2

- At the end of exercise the learner should able to describe and discuss the epidemiological and control measures including the use of essential laboratory tests at the primary care level for communicable diseases. **(CM8.1)**
- Enumerate and describe disease specific National Health Programs including their prevention and treatment of a case. **(CM8.3)**
- Describe and discuss the principles of planning, implementing and evaluating control measures for disease at community level bearing in mind the public health importance of the disease. **(CM8.5)**
- Discuss the role of the child developmental unit in management of developmental delay. **(PE3.5)**
- Visit a child developmental unit and observe its functioning. **(PE3.7)**
- Discuss the principles, the initiation, attributes, frequency, techniques and hygiene related to complementary feeding including IYCF. **(PE8.2)**
- Elicit history on the complementary feeding habits. **(PE8.4)**
- Counsel and educate mothers on the best practices in complementary feeding. **(PE8.5)**
- Describe the age related nutritional needs of infants, children and adolescents including micronutrients and vitamins. **(PE9.1)**
- Describe the tools and methods for assessment and classification of nutritional status of infants, children and adolescents. **(PE9.2)**
- Calculate the age related calorie requirement in Health and disease and identify gap. **(PE9.5)**
- Assess and classify the nutrition status of infants, children and adolescents and recognize deviations. **(PE9.6)**
- Identify children with under nutrition as per IMNCI criteria and plan referral. **(PE10.4)**
- State the vision and outline the goals, strategies and plan of action of NHM and other important national programs pertaining to maternal and child health including RMNCH A+, RBSK, RKSK, JSSK mission Indradhanush and ICDS. **(PE17.1)**
- Explain the components of the universal immunization program and the national immunization program. **(PE19.1)**
- Explain the epidemiology of vaccine preventable diseases. **(PE19.2)**

A 18-month-old child presented to a PHC covering 35,000 populations, with complaints of fever, cough, and conjunctival redness. The child was accompanied by his mother who was illiterate and a daily wage laborer. The birth order of this child was third and he weighed 9 kg and length was 75 cm. His developmental milestones were also delayed. On eliciting the history from the mother, the medical officer in-charge of the PHC found out that rashes appeared four days after the appearance of fever. Rashes started from the face and then spread to the rest of the body. The immunization status of the child was not documented, and mother told she never had any of her children vaccinated. The environmental history revealed that the child came from a slum area and had 6 members residing in 2 rooms, with inadequate ventilation, which suggested overcrowding. Mother also reported that there were two children in her neighborhood who had fever with similar rashes, cough and coryza nearly 10 days back. On examination the rashes were maculo-papular in appearance and the lung fields was bilaterally clear.

- What is the likely diagnosis?
- What should be the management plan?

Guide Notes

- Epidemiology of measles
- Management of measles
- Differential diagnosis of fever with rash
- Viral exanthemas in pediatric age group.

EXERCISE 8.3

- At the end of exercise, the learner should be able to explain the components of the universal immunization program and the national immunization program. **(PE19.1)**
- Explain the epidemiology of vaccine preventable diseases. **(PE19.2)**
- Vaccine description with regard to classification of vaccines, strain used, dose, route, schedule, risks, benefits and side effects, indications and contraindications. **(PE19.3)**
- Define cold chain and discuss the methods of safe storage and handling of vaccines. **(PE19.4)**

A 3-year-old unimmunized boy presented with fever with gradual rise of temperature. He is also suffering from headache, body ache, malaise, and loss of appetite. The child is having pain in the throat and difficulty swallowing. On examination of the throat, his mouth smells foul, a yellowish membrane is visible on tonsils, and surrounding tissue is congested and edematous. On an attempt to peel off the membrane, bleeding occurred. Regional cervical group of lymph nodes are enlarged and tender. The child also has mild toxemia.

- What is the probable diagnosis?
- Discuss the prevention of this disease?

Guide Notes

- Diphtheria
- Primary and Secondary level of prevention in case of diphtheria

EXERCISE 8.4

- At the end of exercise, the learner should be able to explain the components of the universal immunization program and the national immunization program. **(PE19.1)**
- Explain the epidemiology of vaccine preventable diseases. **(PE19.2)**
- Vaccine description with regard to classification of vaccines, strain used, dose, route, schedule, risks, benefits and side effects, indications and contraindications. **(PE19.3)**
- Define cold chain and discuss the methods of safe storage and handling of vaccines. **(PE19.4)**
- Describe the application of interventions at various levels of prevention. **(CM1.5)**

A 3-year-old boy presents with an annoying cough from 3 weeks. The illness started insidiously with fever, dry hacking irritant cough along with malaise and anorexia. After ten days, the cough progressed and became paroxysmal. During paroxysm of cough, there was facial congestion, eyes widened with tears and mouth opens with saliva dropping. A deep high-pitched inspiratory whoop is audible during paroxysm. At the end of the episode, the child vomits, exhausted and go into sleep or another attack of cough.

- What is the probable diagnosis?
- Discuss the epidemiology and prevention of this disease?

Guide Notes

- Pertussis
- Management of pertussis
- Differential diagnoses of pertussis
- Vaccines against pertussis and their place in the NIS.

EXERCISE 8.5

- At the end of exercise, the learner should be able to describe the epidemiological basis of common infectious diseases. **(MI1.3)**
- Discuss and describe the common causes, pathophysiology and manifestations of fever in various regions in India including bacterial, parasitic and viral causes (e.g. dengue, chikungunya, typhus). **(IM4.3)**

A 10-year-old girl presented with fever and chills followed by headache and vomiting. Headache is violent and bursting type. She is resentful, irritable, and uncooperative. After vomiting, the headache increases in intensity. Petechial rashes appeared on skin. On examination, the physician observed stiffness of the neck. Lumbar puncture showed purulent CSF, with elevated opening pressure. Spinal fluid analysis showed decreased glucose and increased protein concentrations. Microscopic examination of CSF reported increased polymorphs. Gram's staining demonstrated gram-negative diplococci.

- What is the probable diagnosis?
- Discuss the epidemiology and prevention of this disease?

Guide Notes

- Meningococcal meningitis
- Meningococcal vaccine
- Kernig and Brudzinski signs
- Compare the bacterial, fungal, viral, and tuberculosis meningitis and draw gross differences.

EXERCISE 8.6

- At the end of exercise, the learner should be able to explain the components of the universal immunization program and the national immunization program. **(PE19.1)**
- Explain the epidemiology of vaccine preventable diseases. **(PE19.2)**
- Vaccine description with regard to classification of vaccines, strain used, dose, route, schedule, risks, benefits and side effects, indications and contraindications. **(PE19.3)**
- Describe the epidemiological basis of common infectious diseases. **(MI1.3)**

An 8-year-old girl presented with painful swelling of both cheeks and surrounding jaw area. She also complained of myalgia, headache, malaise, and low-grade fever. Swelling first appeared in front of the lower part of the ear, later spread to the lower half of the cheeks and jaws. On examination, the angle of the jawbone below the ear is obliterated, bilaterally.

- What is the likely diagnosis?
- Discuss the epidemiology and prevention of this disease?

Guide Notes

- Mumps
- Prevention and complications of mumps
- Vaccines against mumps.

EXERCISE 8.7

- At the end of exercise, the learner should be able to describe the aetiology and basis of water borne diseases /jaundice/hepatitis/diarrheal diseases. **(CM3.3)**
- Define and describe common nutrition related health disorders (including macro-PEM, Micro-iron, Zn, iodine, Vit. A), their control and management. **(CM5.3)**
- Describe Universal Immunization Program; Integrated Management of Neonatal and Childhood Illness (IMNCI) and other existing programs. **(CM10.5)**
- Describe and discuss the following National Health programmes including immunisation, tuberculosis, leprosy, malaria, HIV, filaria, kala azar, diarrhoeal diseases, anaemia and nutritional disorders, blindness, non-communicable diseases, cancer and iodine deficiency. **(PH1.55)**
- Identify children with under nutrition as per IMNCI criteria and plan referral. **(PE10.4)**

During your internship, you've been posted in a PHC during your Community Medicine posting. Suddenly a girl Priya came in your emergency OPD, with diarrhea from the last 4 days. Her age was 2 years and 2 months and weighed 9 kg. She is afebrile and did not show any danger signs such as cough or difficulty in breathing. You enquire about any incidence of passage of blood in stool, to which Priya's mother said no. When you checked for any signs of dehydration, you saw that Priya is conscious but lethargic. She is not irritable and does not have any sign of dehydration such as sunken eyes. On conducting skin pinch test, her skin goes back within 2 seconds.

- Classify this diarrhea according to IMNCI criteria.
- Suggest appropriate treatment plan for Priya.
- What are the important warning signs which a mother should look for and return to the health facility?

Guide Notes

- Diarrhea and dehydration
- IMNCI
- Updated WHO-ORS formulation and role of zinc.

EXERCISE 8.8

- At the end of exercise, the learner should be able to describe the epidemiological basis of common infectious diseases. **(MI1.3)**
- Describe the aetiology and basis of water borne diseases/jaundice/hepatitis/diarrheal diseases. **(CM3.3)**

Aarav is doing his internship from Medical College situated in Bhopal. His PSM posting has started and he is currently posted at an Urban Health Training Centre (UHTC). During his OPD timing, a father of a 9-year-old boy Shashwat, studying in IV Standard in a renowned school of Bhopal city, rushed into his room and told that his son recently developed mild fever, malaise, anorexia, with on and off nausea and diarrhea. He also has abdominal pain with skin rash and complained of dark colored urine and pale/clay colour stool from the last 2 weeks. During clinical examination, Aarav noticed that Shashwat did not have any sign of dehydration but had jaundice. Liver was just palpable on abdominal examination. Shashwat' s diet includes food mostly prepared by his mother at home, except for breakfast and lunch, which is offered by the school during school timings, as informed by his father. Based on the history given by Shashwat's father and the clinical findings, Aarav advised him Liver Function Test (LFT) and stool examination.

- Has Aarav reached his provisional diagnosis? If yes, then what was it?
- Name different serological tests which help him to confirm his diagnosis.
- Do active and passive immunization have significant roles in prevention of this disease?

Guide Notes

- Hepatitis A and E
- Hepatitis prevention and control.

EXERCISE 8.9

- At the end of exercise, the learner should be able to conduct immunization in special situations like-HIV positive children, immunodeficiency, pre-term, organ transplant, those who received blood and blood products, splenectomized children, adolescents and travelers. **(PE19.5)**
- Describe the epidemiological basis of common infectious diseases. **(MI1.3)**

Mohanlal, a 55 years aged male, who lives in Ratlam city, has undergone right knee joint replacement, 3 and a half months back. His surgical record showed that profuse bleeding occurred intraoperatively, and his then hemoglobin was recorded to be 7.5 g/dl. His treating physician immediately decided for blood transfusion (BT) to maintain the normal hemoglobin levels.[2] units of BT after proper grouping and cross matching were arranged and given. During his follow up visit at 6 weeks, the patient had complaints of arthralgia, myalgia, pruritis and Lichen planus like lesions throughout the body. The physician also noticed that the patient was icteric and hence ordered a liver function test. LFT showed increased levels of both direct and indirect bilirubin, SGOT and SGPT.

- Which type of hepatitis is Mohanlal suffering from?
- Is there any role of health education to reduce the incidence/occurence of this disease?
- Name other diseases which have high chances of transmitting through blood transfusion?
- What are the different preventive and control measures you can take to reduce this kind of disease?

Guide Notes

- Hepatitis B and C
- Hepatitis prevention and control
- Compare transmission rates of Hepatitis and HIV.

EXERCISE 8.10

- At the end of this exercise, the learner should be able to describe the epidemiological basis of common infectious diseases. **(MI1.3)**
- Describe the aetiology and basis of water borne diseases/jaundice/hepatitis/diarrheal diseases. **(CM3.3)**

A young lady Meenal 26 years of age living in Mini Metro city, is very fond of eating non-vegetarian and street foods, especially pani-puri, twice in a week. Suddenly one day she developed mild fever, anorexia, nausea and diarrhea, all of which resolved spontaneously after 2–3 days, without any reported complication. After some time, she got pregnant. She went to a health facility for Routine ANC check- up and examination. Her obstetrician asked her about the history of any recent infections, then she shared history of this infection with her doctor. On further questioning, Meenal mentioned passing dark colored urine and pale colored stool, both for 7 days after her condition resolved. The doctor enquired about her eating habits and advised her to restrain from eating street food during the current monsoon season as she is pregnant.

- What could be the provisional diagnosis in this case?
- Is there any relation of pregnant state of the patient and her prior affliction?
- What is Fulminant hepatitis?
- Discuss preventive and containment measures against such kind of infection?

Guide Notes

- Hepatitis E and pregnancy
- Fulminant hepatitis and control measures

EXERCISE 8.11

- At the end of exercise, the learner should be able to describe and discuss the principles of planning, implementing and evaluating control measures for disease at community level bearing in mind the public health importance of the disease. **(CM 8.5)**

A young male comes to the clinic with his 4-year boy. He is concerned that his child is not gaining weight and that his height is also less as compared to his peers. He also reports that his son occasionally has mild fever and coughs out bloody sputum. When the doctor asks about the child's daily routine, he finds out that his son spends most of his time playing in a nearby farmland and has a habit of eating soil and mud. Doctor orders routine blood workup for the child. His peripheral blood picture (PBS) shows anemia and eosinophilia with absolute eosinophil count at 1540 cells/mm^3. The doctor further ordered stool examination.

- Does the above scenario point towards any worm infestation?
- What is Loffler's syndrome?
- What is the other manifestation which could take place after a worm infestation?
- What preventive and control measures can be taken to control this condition?

Guide Notes

- Various ectoparasites and endoparasites which affect humans
- *Worm infection/infestation:* Public health problem
- Manifestations and control measures.

EXERCISE 8.12

- At the end of exercise, the learner should be able to describe and discuss the epidemiological and control measures including the use of essential laboratory tests at the primary care level for communicable diseases. **(CM8.1)**
- Enumerate and describe disease specific National Health Programs including their prevention and treatment of a case. **(CM8.3)**
- Describe and discuss the principles of planning, implementing and evaluating control measures for disease at community level bearing in mind the public health importance of the disease. **(CM8.5)**

Rohit, a 28-year aged male, photographer by profession, recently returned to India after his visit from Sudan. Now after 6 months of his return, he visits the OPD with complaints of blisters and ulceration on his right leg associated with itching and burning, and generalized arthralgia and arthritis. Few days back, in the ulcerated area he reported seeing some worm. He also complains of recent onset allergic manifestations.

- What is your provisional diagnosis?
- Discuss the peripheral blood picture of this patient, if ordered
- Enlist National Health Programme running to eliminate this disease
- Briefly discuss the prevention strategies.

Guide Notes

- Dracunculiasis
- National Guinea Worm Control Programme.

EXERCISE 8.13

- At the end of exercise, the learner should be able to describe and discuss the epidemiological and control measures including the use of essential laboratory tests at the primary care level for communicable diseases. **(CM8.1)**
- Describe and discuss the principles of planning, implementing and evaluating control measures for disease at community level bearing in mind the public health importance of the disease. **(CM8.5)**

A 16-year boy Sourabh came to the OPD with complaints of fever, mild abdominal pain, dysentery, with passage of stool 10-12 times a day, and tenesmus. On enquiring about his dietary habits and living condition, the doctor finds out that his family uses water supplied by municipal corporation of the city which is often contaminated because of leakage in water pipes. The doctor performs an abdominal examination which reveals abdominal tenderness and mild hepatomegaly. Subsequently routine stool examination and hepatic ultrasound was ordered. Stool examination revealed grossly foul-smelling stool, semifluid in consistency and dark brown in colour. Hepatic USG showed a single abscess in the right lobe of the liver.

- What is your provisional diagnosis?
- Discuss public health measures to control this kind of disease?

Guide Notes

- Amoebiasis
- Causes of dysentery.

EXERCISE 8.14

- At the end of exercise, the learner should be able to describe and discuss the epidemiological and control measures including the use of essential laboratory tests at the primary care level for communicable diseases. **(CM8.1)**
- Describe and discuss the principles of planning, implementing and evaluating control measures for disease at community level bearing in mind the public health importance of the disease. **(CM8.5)**
- Describe Universal Immunization Program; Integrated Management of Neonatal and Childhood Illness (IMNCI) and other existing programs. **(CM10.5)**
- Describe the age related nutritional needs of infants, children and adolescents including micronutrients and vitamins. **(PE9.1)**
- Describe the tools and methods for assessment and classification of nutritional status of infants, children and adolescents. **(PE9.2)**
- Identify children with under nutrition as per IMNCI criteria and plan referral. **(PE10.4)**

A 4-year girl Pihu was brought by her mother to the pediatric OPD. Her mother complained that Pihu is having diarrhea with loss of appetite. Pihu is also underweight for her age. They lived in an urban slum area deprived of proper sanitary disposal facility. Doctor ordered stool examination, which revealed grossly bulky stool and microscopic picture of the sample showed lots of fat droplets and looked like this:

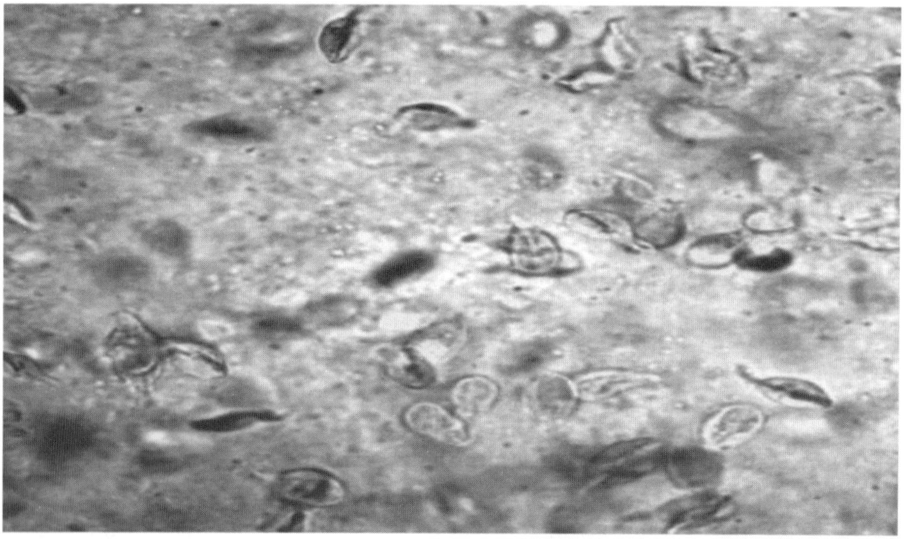

- Interpret the microscopic picture of stool. Identify the protozoa.
- What is the drug of choice for treatment of this acute condition?
- What additional finding will you get on microscopic examination of stool of this patient?
- How will you prevent the spread of this disease within the community?

Guide Notes

- Giardiasis
- Diagnosis, prevention and control.

EXERCISE 8.15

- At the end of exercise, the learner should be able to describe and discuss the epidemiological and control measures including the use of essential laboratory tests at the primary care level for communicable diseases. **(CM8.1)**
- Enumerate and describe disease specific National Health Programs including their prevention and treatment of a case. **(CM8.3)**
- Describe and discuss the principles of planning, implementing and evaluating control measures for disease at community level bearing in mind the public health importance of the disease. **(CM8.5)**
- Describe the epidemiological basis of common infectious diseases. **(MI1.3)**

A 26-years lady who lives in an urban slum of a big city, came with his 1-year-old boy Aarav to attend pediatric OPD. She complained that his child has high fever for the last 3 days and since last night he is having difficulty in moving both of his legs. On further examination, it was found that on its second day, fever was associated with malaise and severe myalgia in the limbs, followed by asymmetrically distributed lower motor neuron (LMN) type of flaccid paralysis without any sensory loss. Careful history taking elicited that Aarav spends most of his time playing in mud just outside their house, after she goes out for work. She mentioned that since their house lacked proper sanitation facilities, they practice open defecation. What is your probable diagnosis?

- Discuss differential diagnoses of flaccid paralysis?
- What are the different public health measures to control this disease?

Guide Notes

- AFP surveillance
- Poliomyelitis.

EXERCISE 8.16

- At the end of exercise, the learner should able to describe Universal Immunization Program; Integrated Management of Neonatal and Childhood Illness (IMNCI) and other existing programs. **(CM10.5)**
- Define the term complementary feeding. **(PE8.1)**
- Discuss the principles, the initiation, attributes, frequency, techniques and hygiene related to complementary feeding including IYCF. **(PE8.2)**
- Enumerate the common complementary foods. **(PE8.3)**
- Elicit history on the complementary feeding habits. **(PE8.4)**
- Counsel and educate mothers on the best practices in complementary feeding. **(PE8.5)**
- Describe the age related nutritional needs of infants, children and adolescents including micronutrients and vitamins. **(PE9.1)**
- Describe the tools and methods for assessment and classification of nutritional status of infants, children and adolescents. **(PE9.2)**
- Calculate the age related calorie requirement in Health and disease and identify gap. **(PE9.5)**
- Assess and classify the nutrition status of infants, children and adolescents and recognize deviations. **(PE9.6)**
- Identify children with under nutrition as per IMNCI criteria and plan referral. **(PE10.4)**

Monu is an eight months boy having weight of 6 kg. He had complaint of diarrhea from last 20 days. He also had some signs of dehydration on general looking. His weight is not normal as with same age child. The doctor further evaluated the history of child by asking more about child so, her mother told that he only takes cow milk and some amount of vegetable. His face is also pale in general looking.

- What is your probable diagnosis?
- Is there any requirement of immediate admission to the child?

- What are key preventive and treatment measures against diarrhea?
- What kind of food he has to take after getting cured?

Guide Notes

- Discuss anthropometric measurements
- Discuss Infant and Young Child Feeding (IYCF) Program
- Discuss importance and advantages of breast feeding.

EXERCISE 8.17

- At the end of exercise, the learner should be able to describe and discuss the following National Health programmes including immunisation, tuberculosis, leprosy, malaria, HIV, filaria, kala azar, diarrhoeal diseases, anaemia and nutritional disorders, blindness, non-communicable diseases, cancer and iodine deficiency. **(PH1.55)**
- State the vision and outline the goals, strategies and plan of action of NHM and other important national programs pertaining to maternal and child health including RMNCH A+, RBSK, RKSK, JSSK mission Indradhanush and ICDS. **(PE17.1)**
- Describe the aetiology and basis of water borne diseases/jaundice/hepatitis/diarrheal diseases. **(CM3.3)**
- Describe Universal Immunization Program; Integrated Management of Neonatal and Childhood Illness (IMNCI) and other existing programs. **(CM10.5)**

One day in a PHC, when you are working as medical officer. Suddenly one day Suresh rushed in an emergency holding his son Mahesh in his arms. His son is four years old and had weight of 15 kg. He is having diarrhea from last 5 days but did not have blood in stool. He is irritable and had sunken eyes as per her mother. You started clinical examination in that you noticed that Mahesh did not have eager to drink. On Skin pinch test, skin goes very slowly more than 2 seconds.

- What is your probable diagnosis?
- According to IMNCI, which plan is most preferred to this child?
- How will you schedule the treatment plan, calculate total fluid required for this child?
- What are key strategies to combat diarrhea?

Guide Notes

- Discuss management of diarrhea in severely malnourished children
- Discuss RMNCH+A
- Discuss the importance of zinc ORS corner.

EXERCISE 8.18

- At the end of exercise, learner should be able to define and describe common nutrition related health disorders (including macro-PEM, Micro-iron, Zn, iodine, Vit. A), their control and management. **(CM5.3)**
- Describe Universal Immunization Program; Integrated Management of Neonatal and Childhood Illness (IMNCI) and other existing programs. **(CM10.5)**

Role play (after setting up an ORS zinc corner by students, in this role play a doctor will teach a mother how to care for a dehydrated child).

REFERENCES

1. Kadri's IAPSM's Textbook of Community Medicine, 2nd edn, pages 246, 250, 256, 291, 295, 299, 319, 330, 332, 333, 340, 348, 413, 419.
2. Park's Textbook of Preventive and Social Medicine Medicine, 26th edn, pages 158, 236, 244, 258, 518, 612, 621.

CHAPTER

9

Non-communicable Diseases

Competency code	*Competency addressed*	*Exercise*
CM2.2	Describe the socio-cultural factors, family (types), its role in health and disease and demonstrate in a simulated environment the correct assessment of socio-economic status	9.7
CM2.4	Describe social psychology, community behavior and community relationship and their impact on health and disease	9.6
CM2.5	Describe poverty and social security measures and its relationship to health and disease	9.7
CM8.2	Describe and discuss the epidemiological and control measures including the use of essential laboratory tests at the primary care level for non-communicable diseases (diabetes, hypertension, stroke, obesity and cancer, etc.)	9.1–9.9
CM15.3	Describe Mental Health Programme	9.10
PS19.1	Describe the relevance, role and status of community psychiatry	9.1
PS19.2	Describe the objectives strategies and contents of the National Mental Health Programme	9.10

EXERCISE 9.1

- At the end of this exercise, you should be able to describe and discuss the epidemiological and control measures including the use of essential laboratory tests at the primary care level for non- communicable diseases (diabetes, hypertension, stroke, obesity and cancer, etc.) **(CM8.2)**
- Describe the relevance, role and status of community psychiatry. **(PS19.1)**

During the community health centre (CHC) posting, you diagnosed a patient with diabetes mellitus. The patient was a 55-year-old female. Her fasting blood sugar was 210 mg/dl, blood pressure was 135/82 mm Hg.

- Which investigations will you order for this patient before starting treatment?
- Discuss the pharmacological interventions for this patient.
- Discuss the non-pharmacological interventions for this patient.
  - Lifestyle modifications (diet and physical activity)
  - Blood sugar monitoring
  - Prevention of complications

Guide Notes

- Diabetes mellitus
- Short-and long-term complications of DM.

EXERCISE 9.2

At the end of this exercise, you should be able to describe and discuss the epidemiological and control measures including the use of essential laboratory tests at the primary care level for non-communicable diseases (diabetes, hypertension, stroke, obesity and cancer etc.) **(CM8.2)**

You are posted at a PHC. During your field visit, you came across a 50-year aged male who wants to get himself and his 47-year aged wife, screened for hypertension.

- Under which programme will you offer them screening for hypertension?
- Under this programme, who should screen these individuals?
- What is the interval of screening, as outlined by this programme?
- What are the eligibility criteria for hypertension screening under the national programme?

Guide Notes

- Different levels of prevention of hypertension
- NPCDCS
- Venn diagram for prevalence of hypertension.

EXERCISE 9.3

At the end of this exercise, you should be able to describe and discuss the epidemiological and control measures including the use of essential laboratory tests at the primary care level for non-communicable diseases (diabetes, hypertension, stroke, obesity and cancer, etc.) **(CM8.2)**

You are posted as an intern at the UHC. A 55-year-old male attended your OPD. His BP was 156/88 mm of Hg, random blood sugar (RBS) was 204 mg/dl and a BMI of 31 kg/m^2. He complained of chronic knee pain which was diagnosed as osteoarthritis (OA)

- Discuss the pharmacological management for this patient.
- Discuss the non-pharmacological interventions for this patient:
  - What dietary advice will you give to this patient?
  - How will you counsel this patient regarding his physical activity?
  - Monitoring of blood pressure and blood sugar

Guide Notes

- Morbidity in the old age group
- Global and national approaches in geriatric healthcare services.

EXERCISE 9.4

At the end of this exercise, you should be able to describe and discuss the epidemiological and control measures including the use of essential laboratory tests at the primary care level for non-communicable diseases (diabetes, hypertension, stroke, obesity and cancer, etc.) **(CM8.2)**

A 35-year-old female, residing in rural area, is having irregular bleeding per vagina since last few weeks. Her neighbor advised her to get screened for cervical cancer.

- Under which national program will she be offered screening?
- Under programmatic conditions, who is supposed to screen this lady for cervical cancer?
- What are the guidelines for cervical cancer screening in India?
    - Eligibility
    - Method of screening
    - Referral chain for diagnosis and management.

Guide Notes

- Common cancers in India
- Screening of cancer in community.

EXERCISE 9.5

At the end of this exercise, you should be able to describe and discuss the epidemiological and control measures including the use of essential laboratory tests at the primary care level for non-communicable diseases (diabetes, hypertension, stroke, obesity and cancer, etc.) **(CM8.2)**

A 47-year-old male resident of village covered under your RHTC, presents with multiple white-colored ulcers of oral mucosa. He is a tobacco chewer and chronic smoker. He is apprehensive and wants to get screened for oral cancer.

- Under which national program, will he be offered screening?
- Under programmatic conditions, who is supposed to screen this person for oral cancer?
- What are the guidelines for oral cancer screening in India?
    - Eligibility criteria
    - Method of screening
    - Referral chain for diagnosis and management.

Guide Note

- DDs for white oral lesions.

EXERCISE 9.6

- At the end of this exercise, you should be able to describe and discuss the epidemiological and control measures including the use of essential laboratory tests at the primary care level for non-communicable diseases (diabetes, hypertension, stroke, obesity and cancer, etc.) **(CM8.2)**
- Describe social psychology, community behavior and community relationship and their impact on health and disease. **(CM2.4)**

A 53-year-old male visited your OPD with complaints of fever, cough, and cold. On general examination, it was noted that the patient was obese. His weight and height were 90 kg and 160 cm, respectively. The patient has a desk job and a sedentary lifestyle and lives in a very crowded area.

- Which investigations will you advise this patient keeping in mind the obesity and sedentary lifestyle of the patient?
- Discuss the diet plan of this patient.
- What advice will you give this patient regarding physical activity?

Guide Notes

- Other clinical findings in hyperlipidemia
- Obesity
- Methods of Nutritional assessment.

EXERCISE 9.7

- At the end of this exercise, you should be able to describe the socio-cultural factors, family (types), its role in health and disease and demonstrate in a simulated environment the correct assessment of socio-economic status. **(CM2.2)**
- Enumerate poverty and social security measures and its relationship to health and disease. **(CM2.5)**
- Describe and discuss the epidemiological and control measures including the use of essential laboratory tests at the primary care level for non-communicable diseases (diabetes, hypertension, stroke, obesity and cancer, etc.) **(CM8.2)**

You are posted as a resident at a PHC. During your field visit, a 40-year-old female came to you with complain of productive cough since last 2 months. There was no history of fever, blood in sputum, and contact with any TB patient. She has been using *chulha* for cooking for many years. Her husband is a chronic smoker and frequently smokes indoors at home. There are two children in the family, a 15-year-old boy and a 12-year-girl.

- What is your provisional diagnosis?
- Based on the negative findings, which differential diagnoses did you rule out?
- What investigations will you order for confirming the diagnosis?
- What preventive measures will you advise her to halt the progression of her condition?
    - At individual level
    - At family level
    - At household level.

Guide Notes

- Epidemiology of COPD
- Prevention and Control of COPD and related diseases.

EXERCISE 9.8

At the end of this exercise describe and discuss the epidemiological and control measures including the use of essential laboratory tests at the primary care level for non-communicable diseases (diabetes, hypertension, stroke, obesity and cancer, etc.) **(CM8.2)**

You are posted as an intern at UHTC. During your field visit, you visited a family, with recently diagnosed case of NAFLD. The patient is a 42-year-female and is working as a data entry operator. She is taking treatment from district hospital (DH).

- What advice will you give her regarding her treatment?
- How will you counsel her family members regarding the prognosis of disease?
- What is the programme under which this disease will be managed?

Guide Notes

- NAFLD: Epidemiology, types, and treatment rationale
- NP-NCD.

EXERCISE 9.9

At the end of this exercise you should be able to describe and discuss the epidemiological and control measures including the use of essential laboratory tests at the primary care level for non-communicable diseases (diabetes, hypertension, stroke, obesity and cancer, etc.) **(CM8.2)**

While travelling to your RHTC, you notice an moving vehicle accident between a two-wheeler and a heavy motor vehicle. The heavy motor vehicle fled away, and the two-wheeler occupant was in semi-conscious condition, having sustained multiple bruises all over the body.

- With reference to the above scenario, what is expected of you at the RTA scene?
- Briefly describe the pre-hospital treatment in this case.
- Explain the pre-event, event, and post-event phases in accidentology?

Guide Notes

- Haddon's matrix
- Epidemiology of accidents.

EXERCISE 9.10

- At the end of this exercise, you should be able to describe Mental Health Programme. **(CM15.3)**
- Enumerate the objectives strategies and contents of the National Mental Health Programme. **(PS19.2)**

Tausheed, 63-years-old, a widower, resident of Ormanjhi, was brought to your RHTC OPD, by his younger brother Zaid. Zaid informed that Tausheed has been showing some behavioral changes since the past 4–5 weeks. He has become suspicious about every activity and person around him, with frequents bouts of aggressive outbursts. He is experiencing sleeplessness and decreased appetite for the past 20–25 days. Zaid also informs that apart from the suspiciousness, he is reluctant to attend any kind of social gathering and prefers to be left alone in his room, where he lies down throughout the day, only getting to have his meals. His behavior is quite salty, and he always walks with his hands on the back, complaining about generalized body ache, more at neck and lower back. Tausheed was conscious and well-oriented at the time of presentation but kept on abusing his younger brother since he was brought here against her will. The interns at RHTC took Tausheed to a separate room, for clinical examination, during which Zaid mentioned that Tausheed had been aggressive since the beginning, but his paranoid behavior and body aches started gradually since his wife, passed away 5 months back. He has 2 sons, both married and live with him in the same household.

- What according to you could be the provisional diagnosis in this case?
- What should be the appropriate next step as the PG-on-duty at the RHTC?
- What crucial information did the interns and PG-on-duty missed to elicit?

Guide Notes

- Features of a mentally healthy person and warning signals of poor mental health
- NMHP.
- ICD-10 and DSM-V classification of mental disorders.
- Substance use and dependence.
- Comprehensive mental health action plan 2013–2030.

REFERENCES

1. Kadri's IAPSM's textbook of Community Medicine. 2nd edn, pages 487, 496, 506, 514, 529, 531, 543, 544, 579, 648, 651, 893, 916.
2. Park's Textbook of Preventive and Social Medicine. 26th edn, pages 419, 427, 438, 443, 447, 451, 453, 528.
3. Purushottam Giri-Epidemiology and Programmatic Management of NCDs in India. 1st edn. 2023 pages 01–199.

FURTHER READING

1. Dietary guidelines for Indians: A manual. National Institute of Nutrition. Hyderabad.
2. Operational Framework: Management of Common Cancers. Ministry of Health and Family Welfare. Government of India.
3. Training Module for Medical Officers for Prevention, Control and Population Level Screening of Hypertension, Diabetes and Common Cancer (Oral, Breast and Cervical).

CHAPTER

10

Nutrition

Competency code	Competency addressed	Exercise
CM5.1	Describe the common sources of various nutrients and special nutritional requirements according to age, sex, activity, physiological conditions	10.6–10.9
CM5.2	Describe and demonstrate the correct method of performing a nutritional assessment of individuals, families and the community by using the appropriate method	10.20
CM5.3	Define and describe common nutrition related health disorders (including macro-PEM, micro-iron, Zn, iodine, vit. A), their control and management.	10.7, 10.11, 10.12, 10.14–10.16, 10.18
CM5.5	Describe the methods of nutritional surveillance, principles of nutritional education and rehabilitation in the context of sociocultural factors.	10.17
CM5.7	Describe food hygiene	10.10
CM5.8	Describe and discuss the importance and methods of food fortification and effects of additives and adulteration	10.1–10.5, 10.19
CM10.3	Describe local customs and practices during pregnancy, childbirth, lactation and child feeding practices	10.13
IM9.15	Describe the national programs for anemia prevention	10.15
PE8.1	Define the term complementary feeding	10.13
PE8.2	Discuss the principles the initiation, attributes, frequency, techniques and hygiene related to complementary feeding	10.13

EXERCISE 10.1

At the end of this exercise, you should be able to describe and discuss the importance and methods of food fortification and effects of additives and adulteration. **(CM5.8)**

A medical officer in Punjab during his posting in a PHC came across an unusual outbreak of gastroenteritis, involving many families. All of them presented with diarrhea, vomiting, and bilateral pitting edema with tenderness over the edematous part and erythematous rash all over the body. Some of the family members complained of visual disturbance also. Socio-demographic details showed that they all belonged to a low socioeconomic class and were agricultural laborers by profession. Dietary history revealed that all of them used mustard oil for cooking. From the details of the case history described above,

- What is the probable diagnosis of the outbreak in that community?
- What are the typical signs and symptoms of the condition?
- What is the etio-pathogenesis of the disease?
- What are the preventive and control measures?

Guide Notes

- Adulteration
- Epidemic dropsy
- Investigation of an epidemic outbreak.

EXERCISE 10.2

At the end of this exercise, you should be able to describe and discuss the importance and methods of food fortification and effects of additives and adulteration. **(CM5.8)**

A shopkeeper sells food material at a very low cost to the poor, migrant population of a slum area. He mixes mud and grits to wheat and rice, and lead chromate powder to turmeric powder so that the food material becomes affordable to the poor people and he himself does not incur losses.

- Explain the problem that this community is facing.
- Name the legal act passed by the Indian Parliament to prevent such deceptive practices and protect the consumers.
- How are such practices punished legally?
- Name some food standards followed in India.

Guide Notes

- Prevention of Food Adulteration Act
- Food Toxicants
- Prevention and Control of Food Adulteration in India.

EXERCISE 10.3

At the end of this exercise you should be able to describe and discuss the importance and methods of food fortification and effects of additives and adulteration. **(CM5.8)**

In some tribal villages of Uttar Pradesh and Bihar, it was found that the majority of the adult population had complaints of difficulty while walking. On clinical examination, it was found that most of them had spastic paralysis (mild to severe) and needed support of one or two sticks for walking. On further investigation and questioning, it was found that this group of population consumed *khesari dal* in high amounts for prolonged periods of time because of its low cost.

- With respect to the above given information and details, froman epidemiological point of view, write down the probable diagnosis of the condition.
- Write down the problem statement and agent responsible for this condition.
- What are the different interventions required to prevent this situation?

Guide Notes

- Lathyrism
- Food additives, food fortification and food adulteration.

EXERCISE 10.4

At the end of this exercise you should be able to describe and discuss the importance and methods of food fortification and effects of additives and adulteration. **(CM5.8)**

Due to heavy rains, huge stocks of cereals (wheat and rice) were kept in the marketing yard. These goods were left unattended for nearly two to three months. Stake holders were worried about the safety and quality of the product since humidity and temperature, both were much more in the storage area. The marketing manager wanted to sell these cereals at low cost.

- Which type of toxin would be released if the cereals were infected because of increased temperature and humidity?
- What are the adverse health effects of this toxin on the consumers?

Guide Notes

- Aflatoxin
- Quality assurance and quality control.

EXERCISE 10.5

At the end of this exercise you should be able to describe and discuss the importance and methods of food fortification and effects of additives and adulteration. **(CM5.8)**

As a medical officer in the team of outbreak investigation in a rural area wheres majority of population having agriculture as their occupation, you observed that members of many families presented with symptoms of nausea, vomiting, diarrhea, and cramps in limbs. Few elderly patients had presented with loss of sensation along with gangrene. Detailed history-taking revealed that their staple diet was *bajra*. On visiting the fields, it was seen that there were small black-colored masses and depositions present in between the crops of *bajra*. The farmers worked in those fields and consumed the *bajra* they cultivated.

- Interpret the condition in the face of the details given above.
- What was responsible for this outbreak?
- Suggest measures to Prevent and control this condition so that such episodes don't recur.

Guide Notes

- Ergotism
- Food-borne Diseases
- Food Standards

EXERCISE 10.6

At the end of this exercise, you should be able to describe the common sources of various nutrients and special nutritional requirements according to age, sex, activity, physiological conditions. **(CM5.1)**

A batch of 12 students was posted in Primary Health Centre (PHC), Bhalej, during their Community Medicine (PSM) posting. The students were divided into four groups and each group worked at the sub-centres (SC), where they took part in maternal health checkup under Janani Suraksha Yojana (JSY). At the end of their monthly posting, they analyzed their work and found out that majority of the women were engaged in household work, while some had to do heavy manual labour on daily wages and very few had a sedentary lifestyle due to their office work. They also found that anemia was seen in many women, along with pedal oedema. Some of them complained of weight gain and weighed more than recommended for their age.

- Mention energy requirements for the females in the different type of working category, mentioned above i.e., heavy work, moderate and sedentary.
- What should be the energy requirement of women during pregnancy and lactation in addition to the normal requirements?
- Recommend appropriate diet according to their dietary requirement based on the respective work group they belong to.

Guide Notes

- RDA
- Balanced diet and prudent diet.

EXERCISE 10.7

- At the end of this exercise, you should be able to describe the common sources of various nutrients and special nutritional requirements according to age, sex, activity, physiological conditions. **(CM5.1)**
- Define and describe common nutrition related health disorders (including macro-PEM, micro-iron, Zn, iodine, vit. A), their control and management. **(CM5.3)**

You visit a primary school classroom of 3rd standard in a rural area as a part of the School Health Programme (SHP) during your community medicine posting. You see teachers and a medical officer examining students as a part of the programme. The School Health Programme (SHP) was launched to address the health needs of children and adolescents, aged 6–18 years, in government and government-aided schools. It includes Rashtriya Bal Shishu Karyakram (RBSK), Mid-day Meal (MDM) Program, mass deworming, weekly supply of IFA, vitamin A and fortified iodized salt while preparing MDMs. Other interventions included health and nutritional education and providing screening and remedial measures.

- What are the different screening techniques used to identify health problems in children?
- Which health problems are screened during school health check-up?
- Suppose a child is found to have reduced vision, what will be your next step?
- Many children complained of chronic abdominal pain, what is your advice and treatment?

Guide Notes

- School Health Program (SHP)
- IMNCI.

EXERCISE 10.8

At the end of this exercise, you should be able to describe the common sources of various nutrients and special nutritional requirements according to age, sex, activity, physiological conditions. **(CM5.1)**

As a part of field visit in your community medicine posting, on a visit to a small district in Himachal Pradesh, you come across many people including children, with enlarged neck. Some children had very low IQ as well as short stature. Many females gave history of miscarriages.

- Interpret the findings of the field visit and diagnose the condition.
- What is the deficient nutrient that has led to the condition mentioned above and mention the daily requirement of the nutrient in males, females (in non-pregnant and pregnant states) and children?

- What are the components under the National Nutritional Programmes for prevention and control of this condition?
- What are the epidemiological criteria for assessing severity of the disease condition?

Guide Notes

- Nutritional deficiency disorders
- Food pyramid

EXERCISE 10.9

At the end of this exercise, you should be able to describe the common sources of various nutrients and special nutritional requirements according to age, sex, activity, physiological conditions. **(CM5.1)**

A married couple along with their 3-year-old child visits a family health physician. They complain of muscle weakness and bone pain. The wife is a homemaker, and husband is an IT professional working from home. They also describe that 3-year-old frequently complains of aches and pain in lower limbs and wakes up from sleep. As an intern posted in that centre you have to advice the family.

- Which is the nutritional deficiency leading to the type of condition described?
- What is the recommended dietary allowance (RDA) of the nutrient in question for different age groups?
- What is the source and function of that nutrient?
- How will you prevent this condition in future?

Guide Notes

- Vitamin D deficiency and its prevention
- Hypervitaminosis D.

EXERCISE 10.10

At the end of this exercise, you should be able to describe food hygiene. **(CM5.7)**

As part of a routine visit, you are visiting the urban health training centre (UHTC) as a medical officer. Out of the 30 children who consumed mid-day meal at a Govt. Higher primary school, surendranagar, 20 children were brought to the urban health centre with complaints of abdominal pain and vomiting. A similar concern about the quality of food being served in the school had been raised by many parents in the past.

- As a medical officer how would you go about investigating the concerned situation?
- Which is the Implementing agency responsible for the mid-day meal (MDM) scheme?
- How is the supervision and monitoring done to assess the efficiency of the implementation of the scheme at local, district and state levels?
- What measures would you suggest to the teachers to improve the quality of nutrition to children as part of MDM program?
- What steps would you suggest ensuring better coordination among health department and education department?

Guide Notes

- Mid-day Meal Scheme
- Mid-day Meal Programme
- PM-POSHAN

EXERCISE 10.11

At the end of this exercise, you should be able to define and describe common nutrition related health disorders (including macro-PEM, Micro-iron, Zn, iodine, vit. A), their control and management. **(CM5.3)**

As a medical officer you were asked to examine a full term 3-year-old girl. She had no congenital anomalies. Her body weight was found to be11 kg which was less than 2 Z score as per WHO standards, and height was 87 cm. She shows dependent edema of the lower extremities as well as an enlarged abdomen. Her skin shows flaking, irregular depigmentation, hyperpigmentation, and patchy desquamation.

- These findings are most suggestive of which nutritional problems?
- Calculate the energy requirement per day for this child?
- What dietary advice will you give to the mother, for the child?
- What other advice will you give to the mother, for the child?

Guide Notes

- Discuss clinical features of protein energy malnutrition (PEM).
- Discuss calorie and protein requirements according to gender and age.
- Discuss protein and energy rich food advice to be given to mothers, for children.
- Discuss hygiene and immunization advice considering 'The vicious cycle of malnutrition'.
- Differential diagnoses for PEM.

EXERCISE 10.12

At the end of this exercise, you should be able to define and describe common nutrition related health disorders (including macro-PEM, micro-iron, Zn, iodine, vit. A), their control and management. **(CM5.3)**

A clinical study was conducted to assess the factors affecting dietary iron metabolism in adults. It is observed that intestinal absorption of iron can be increased in patients with iron deficiency anemia (IDA) by adding another nutrient to their diet.

- Which nutrient is being suggested by the study, for enhancing iron absorption from diet?
- What are the clinical features of deficiency of the above-mentioned vitamin?
- Enumerate the dietary sources of this vitamin.
- What other dietary advice will you give to a patient with IDA?

Guide Notes

- Discuss clinical features of vitamin C deficiency.
- Discuss promoters and inhibitors of iron absorption.
- Discuss about foods rich in vitamin C and iron.

EXERCISE 10.13

- At the end of this exercise, you should be able to describe local customs and practices during pregnancy, childbirth, lactation and child feeding practices. **(CM10.3)**
- Define the term complementary feeding **(PE8.1)**
- Discuss the principles the initiation, attributes, frequency, techniques and hygiene related to complementary feeding. **(PE8.2)**

Neha Batra is an exclusively breastfed 5-month-old girl. Her weight is 6 kilograms, and length measured as 50 cm. In your clinic, Mrs Batra tells the nurse that if she returns to full-time work in about a week, she may stop breastfeeding her daughter. Mrs Batra asks if she should start feeding infant formula and solid foods to Neha. Mrs Batra is worried that her baby could have adverse reactions when it comes to trying too many new things. She even worries about Neha choking on food. All this was communicated to you indirectly by your nurse.

- What screening would you conduct for Neha?
- Identify three areas of counseling that you would provide to the mother?
- Comment on expressed breast milk and its storage.

Guide Notes

- Growth charting for the child
- Discuss and compare exclusive breastfeeding (EBF), complementary feeding and cow milk feeding
- Breast milk expression and its storage.

EXERCISE 10.14

At the end of this exercise, you should be able to define and describe common nutrition related health disorders (including macro-PEM, micro-iron, Zn, iodine, vit. A), their control and management. **(CM5.3)**

You met your 40-year-old aunt from South America in a marriage. She told you that over the past 2-years she has developed redness and roughness of skin in the sun-exposed areas. She is also suffering from watery diarrhea. Upon physical examination, she exhibited memory loss with confusion. She used multiple ointments for her skin condition, but without relief. She informed you that she eats only home-made fresh food.

- These findings are most suggestive of which vitamin deficiency?
- This is common in people who obtain most of their food energy from corn. Explain why?
- What advice will you give to your aunt?

Guide Notes

- Clinical features of vitamin B_3 deficiency.
- RDA and food items rich in vitamin B_3.

EXERCISE 10.15

- At the end of this exercise, you should be able to define and describe common nutrition related health disorders (including macro-PEM, micro-iron, Zn, iodine, vit. A), their control and management. **(CM5.3)**
- Describe the national programs for anemia prevention. **(IM9.15)**

You are a Medical Officer posted at a PHC. You asked an intern to study a 30-year-old primigravida, who is currently in the 8th month of her gestation. She belongs to a joint family and on using Pareek scale, she fell in the lower socioeconomic status (SES). She experiences increased fatigue and weakness. Laboratory test includes CBC showing Hb to be 8.7 g/dl, Hct around 27.8%, MCV 65 fl, platelet count of 278,000/µl, and TLC around 6500/µl. The RBCs exhibit increased variability in size (anisocytosis) and shape (poikilocytosis) on PBS, with majority being hypochromic and microcytic.

- These findings are most suggestive of which nutrient deficiency?

- What other age groups will you check for above nutrient deficiency under the National Health Program (NHP)?
- What are the strategies to combat the above ailment under the National Health Program?
- What is the recommended prophylactic dose for the above nutrient?

Guide Notes

- Clinical and laboratory features of IDA
- 6*6*6 strategy under Anemia Mukt Bharat
- Prophylactic iron and folic acid dosage for different age groups.

EXERCISE 10.16

At the end of this exercise, you should be able to define and describe common nutrition related health disorders (including macro-PEM, micro-iron, Zn, iodine, vit. A), their control and management. **(CM5.3)**

Your hospital security guard is a 41-year-old man. He complains to you that he has been experiencing progressive dyspnea for the past one year. On auscultation, diffuse crackles are heard at the lung bases bilaterally. His chest X-ray shows pulmonary edema and cardiomegaly. Echocardiography indicates a 45% ejection fraction (EF). Laboratory tests indicate a hemoglobin of 13.6 g/dl, hematocrit 410.5%, and TLC around 6720/µl.

- Which vitamin deficiency is most likely to produce these results?
- What is another form of presentation of the above vitamin deficiency?
- What dietary advice will you give to this person?

Guide Notes

- Discuss clinical features of vitamin B_1 deficiency
- Discuss dry and wet beri-beri
- Discuss about RDA and food items rich in vitamin B_{10}.

EXERCISE 10.17

At the end of this exercise, you should be able to describe the methods of nutritional surveillance, principles of nutritional education and rehabilitation in the context of sociocultural factors. **(CM5.5)**

You are a public health consultant. You were designing a dietary study to assess hypertension and its risks factors. While reviewing the literature, you found that increased dietary sodium consumption was observed to be correlated with increased blood pressure. During the study, an old lady of 65, a known hypertensive for 10 years, on treatment with tab. amlodipine 5 mg OD and was non diabetic asked you the following questions:

- What is the recommendation for dietary salt consumption for her?
- What advice will you give to this old lady to reduce salt consumption at home?
- What is a DASH diet?

Guide Notes

- Dietary guidelines for salt and sodium.
- Hypertensive diet.
- Venn diagram for prevalence of hypertension

EXERCISE 10.18

At the end of this exercise, you should be able to define and describe common nutrition related health disorders (including macro-PEM, micro-iron, Zn, iodine, vit. A), their control and management. **(CM5.3)**

You are a Medical Officer at a PHC and have been invited by the primary school principal for the annual day celebration. There is a mother of Ms. Khushi, 5-year-old child complains that her daughter has developed gradual loss of vision over the past 2-years during nighttime. She was worried whether her daughter would require spectacles. On examination you found there is corneal xerosis.

- This child's vision is most likely to have been prevented by adequate dietary intake of which vitamin?
- What is the recommendation for prophylaxis to prevent this vitamin deficiency in under-five children?
- What therapeutic dosage of the above vitamin will you give to this child?
- What are the dietary sources for the above vitamin to be supplemented in the diet?

Guide Notes

- Clinical features of vitamin A deficiency and its prevention
- Vitamin A prophylaxis as per National Immunization Schedule (NIS).

EXERCISE 10.19

At the end of this exercise, you should be able to describe and discuss the importance and methods of food fortification and effects of additives and adulteration. **(CM5.8)**

You are travelling on a cruise with your friends. Your friend Mr. Kumar complains to you about his 7-year-old son's increasing yellowish discoloration of teeth. You told him to get a consultation done from the dentist. On returning home to Andhra Pradesh, Mr. Kumar visited a dentist with his son. The dentist told Mr Kumar that the yellowish discoloration of his son's teeth is due to fluorosis. That evening Mr Kumar called you to share the dentist's diagnosis. You were discussing with Mr Kumar that World Health Organization has published guidance to control fluoride exposures to establish the important balance between caries prevention and protection against adverse effects. Mr Kumar then asks you the following:

- What is the drinking water standard for fluoride?
- What are the effects of excess levels of fluoride?
- Are there methods that Mr Kumar can use to remove fluoride from my drinking water at home?

Guide Notes

- Discuss drinking water standards
- Discuss effects of excess levels of fluoride in drinking water
- Discuss the methods of de-fluorination of water at household level
- Hard water.

EXERCISE 10.20

At the end of this exercise, you should be able to describe and demonstrate the correct method of performing a nutritional assessment of individuals, families and the community by using the appropriate method. **(CM5.2)**

Growth chart, used for the early identification of growth faltering and under-nutrition is included in the postnatal care section of Mother and Child Protection Card. The growth chart is a plot with age on the X-axis and weight on the Y-axis. It can be plotted only for the child from birth to 5-years of age and weighing, up to 22 kg of weight. Kanha is a 2-year-old male child who visits Anganwadi, Surendranagar with his mother Lakshmi every month to collect ready-to-eat food. On weighing the child, Anganwadi teacher records Kanha's weight to be 9 kg, when she plots the weight of Kanha on growth chart, she observes it is in yellow zone now. His weight was 9.5 kg last month and was in the green zone.

- What measures should be taken by Anganwadi teacher to ensure healthy weight gain by Kanha?
- What should be conveyed to Lakshmi about Kanha's nutritional status?
- What advise should be given to Lakshmi about Kanha's diet?

Guide Notes

- Growth chart
- Assessment of nutritional status.

REFERENCES

1. Kadri's IAPSM. Textbook of Community Medicine, 2nd edition, pages 26, 28, 31, 45, 47.
2. Park's Textbook of Preventive and Social Medicine. 26th edition, pages 136, 376, 491, 495, 511, 520, 612, 621, 644, 663, 705-710, 726-728, 746-748, 751, 986.

FURTHER READING

1. Anemia Mukt Bharat. Available from https://anemiamuktbharat.info/wp-content/uploads/2019/11/English_Anemia-Mukt-Bharat-Training-Modules-Folder_Lowress.pdf.
2. Growth Monitoring Manual, National Institute of Public Cooperation and Child Development 96, 67–70.
3. Operational framework Weekly Iron Folic Acid Supplementation (WIFS) for adolescent by GOI. Available from: (https://nhm.gov.in/images/pdf/programmes/wifs/operational-framework-wifs/operational_framework_wifs.pdf).
4. WHO. Water and sanitation. Fluorosis Available from: https://www.who.int/water_sanitation_health/diseases-risks/diseases/fluorosis/en/

CHAPTER

11

Maternal and Child Health

Competency code	Competency addressed	Exercise
CM10.1	Describe the current status of reproductive, maternal, newborn and child health	11.1–11,4, 11,7– 11.9
CM10.2	Enumerate and describe the methods of screening high risk groups and common health problems	11.12, 11.13, 11.17, 11.18, 11.20
CM10.3	Describe local customs and practices during pregnancy, childbirth, lactation and child feeding practices	11.9–11.11
CM10.4	Describe the reproductive, maternal, newbornand child health (RMCH); child survival and safe motherhood interventions	11.14–11.16, 11.19
CM10.5	Describe Universal Immunization Program; Integrated Management of Neonatal and Childhood Illness (IMNCI) and other existing programs.	11.9
CM10.6	Enumerate and describe various family planning methods, their advantages and shortcomings	11.6
CM10.7	Enumerate and describe the basis and principles of the Family Welfare Program including the organization, technical and operational aspects	11.5
CM 10.8	Describe the physiology, clinical management and principles of adolescent health including ARSH	11.21
OG1.1	Define and discuss birth rate, maternal mortality and morbidity	11.1

EXERCISE 11.1

At the end of this exercise you should be able to describe the current status of reproductive, maternal, newborn and child health. **(CM10.1)**
Define and discuss birth rate, maternal mortality and morbidity. **(OG1.1)**

A new medical officer in-charge joined a PHC in 2018. He was interested in knowing about some fertility indicators in his area. His health manager gave the data for the year 2017 as follows:

- Mid-year population: 25,700
- Mid-year population of women in 15–49 years' age group: 6,340
- Number of live births: 328.

- Calculate the crude birth rate (CBR) and general fertility rate (GFR) for this given area.
- Which indicator is better among the above two and why?

Guide Notes

- CSSM, MCH
- Fertility indices
- Indices of mortality and morbidity in under-5 children
- RCH, RMNCH+A, RMNCAH+N.

EXERCISE 11.2

At the end of this exercise you should be able to describe the current status of reproductive, maternal, newborn and child health. **(CM10.1)**

An intern posted in RHTC of a medical college was given some fertility related data for a district. The community medicine department asked him to calculate some fertility indicators based upon that data so that it can be used in 'Community Awareness Program on Family Planning' in that district. The data given to him are as follows:

Age group	*ASFR*	*ASMFR*
15–19	29.1	287.5
20–24	176.5	310.9
25–29	152.2	198.2
30–34	57.3	64.2
35–39	19.5	21.1
40–44	5.2	5.7
45–49	1.5	1.6

- Calculate total fertility rate (TFR) and total marital fertility rate (TMFR).
- Which among two indices tell us about an approximate magnitude of completed family size.

Guide Notes

- NSSK, JSSK, JSY, BFHI
- RCH, RMNCH+A, RMNCAH+N
- TFR, TMFR.

EXERCISE 11.3

At the end of this exercise you should be able to describe the current status of reproductive, maternal, newborn and child health. **(CM10.1)**

In the Ramgarh district of Jharkhand, for the year 2019, midyear population of females in the 20–24 years age group in rural and urban areas were 24,300 and16,600, respectively. In the same age group, number of married females in rural and urban areas were 21,800 and 13,500 respectively. The total number of live births in that year was 5600 and 3200 in rural and urban areas respectively.

- Calculate age specific fertility rate (ASFR) and age specific marital fertility rate (ASMFR) in both rural and urban areas for the given age.
- Interpret the differences in ASFR and ASMFR.
- What could be the possible reasons for differences in these indices between rural and urban areas?

Guide Notes

- ASFR, ASMFR
- MCH in SDG.

EXERCISE 11.4

At the end of this exercise you should be able to describe the current status of reproductive, maternal, newborn and child health. **(CM10.1)**

As per fertility statistics in India for the year 2012, age-specific fertility rate (ASFR) in the 15–19 years age group in rural area was 36.3 per 1000 live-births and age-specific marital fertility rate (ASMFR) in the same age group in rural area was 273.8 per 1000 live-births. Similarly, ASFR and ASMFR in the 30–34 years age group in rural area was 68.3 per 1000 live-births and 72.9 per 1000 live-births, respectively.

- Explain the differences between both rates with respect to different age groups.

Guide Notes

- Fertility indices.

EXERCISE 11.5

At the end of this exercise you should be able to enumerate and describe the basis and principles of the Family Welfare Program including the organization, technical and operational aspects. **(CM 10.7)**

A new oral contraceptive, namely 'Suraksha' was given to 500 Eligible Couples for a continuous period of three years. During this same period, 30 women became pregnant despite using 'Suraksha'.

- What is the efficacy of this new oral contraceptive?

Guide Notes

- Eligible couple, target couple
- Unmet needs of contraception
- Failure rates of various contraceptives.

EXERCISE 11.6

At the end of this exercise, you should be able to enumerate and describe various family planning methods, their advantages and shortcomings. **(CM10.6)**

Undergraduate medical students were taken to a health sub-centre for their visit during the 5th semester. Students asked the ANM about eligible couples and contraceptives used by them. ANM gave the following data:

- Number of eligible couples = 800
- IUCD users = 70
- OCP users = 100
- Condom users = 50
- Sterilization done = 120

Assist the students in calculating the couple protection rate (CPR) and effective couple protection rate (ECPR).

Guide Notes

- Couple protection rate (CPR), effective couple protection rate (ECPR)
- Eligible couple, target couple
- Unmet needs of contraception.

EXERCISE 11.7

At the end of this exercise you should be able to describe the current status of reproductive, maternal, newborn and child health. **(CM10.1)**

In 2018, the total population of a district was 567,000. During the same year, 28,000 live births and 63 maternal deaths were recorded in the same area. Also, infants' deaths were reported to be 328 fromthe same district in that year.

- Calculate maternal mortality ratio (MMR)
- Calculate infant mortality rate (IMR)
- List the common causes of maternal and infant mortality in India.

Guide Notes

- Direct and indirect causes of maternal mortality
- Infant mortality rate (IMR)
- Maternal mortality ratio (MMR)
- MDSR.

EXERCISE 11.8

At the end of this exercise you should be able to describe the current status of reproductive, maternal, newborn and child health. **(CM10.1)**

Medical students were taken to a community health centre, covering 128,000 populations in the year 2019. The in-charge of that CHC was asked to provide some data regarding the infant population of that area, to aid the students in conducting exercises related to infant mortality. Following data were given for the year 2019.

- Total live births = 6440
- Death of neonates within 7 days of birth = 40
- Death of neonates within 28 days of birth = 68
- Death of infants between 28 days and one year of age = 30

- Calculate early neonatal mortality rate
- Calculate neonatal mortality rate (NMR)
- Calculate post-neonatal mortality rate
- Calculate infant mortality rate (IMR)
- What do you interpret from the values of these mortality indices?

Guide Notes

- Direct and indirect causes of maternal mortality
- Early neonatal mortality rate
- Infant mortality rate (IMR)
- Neonatal mortality rate (NMR)
- Post-neonatal mortality rate.

EXERCISE 11.9

At the end of this exercise you should be able to describe the current status of reproductive, maternal, newborn and child health. **(CM 10.1)**

Describe local customs and practices during pregnancy, childbirth, lactation and child feeding practices. **(CM 10.3)**

Describe Universal Immunization Program (UIP); Integrated Management of Neonatal and Childhood Illness (IMNCI) and other existing programs. **(CM 10.5)**

A large number of stillbirths were reported by some local newspaper in a district in the year 2011. District health officials sought help from the community medicine department of a nearby government medical college to get exact data on this matter. Postgraduate students were assigned the job and the following data was gathered within a fortnight:

- Mid-year population in 2016 = 644000
- No. of stillbirths in that year = 21
- Total live births in that year = 5390
- Early neonatal deaths in that year = 86

Now,

- Calculate stillbirth rate (SBR).
- Calculate perinatal mortality rate (PMR).
- What is the importance of perinatal mortality rate?

Guide Notes

- Perinatal mortality rate (PMR).
- RCH, RMNCH+A, RMNCAH+N
- Steps under IMNCI
- Stillbirth Rate (SBR).

EXERCISE 11.10

At the end of this exercise, you should be able to describe local customs and practices during pregnancy, childbirth, lactation and child feeding practices. **(CM 10.3)**

An NGO was interested in working for under-5 children in Jharkhand. After discussion, the health officials asked them to work in a district that had considerable geographical difficulties and an inadequate health care delivery system. After reaching the district headquarters, the NGO workers asked for data related to child mortality in that area for the past one year. The following data was given:

- Mid-year population = 327,480
- Total live birth in last one year = 4356
- Total number of under-5 children death = 127.

- Calculate under-5 mortality rate (U5MR)
- Calculate child survival rate. What is its significance?

Guide Notes

- CSSM, MCH, RCH
- Indices of mortality and morbidity in under-5 children
- IYCF
- Steps under IMNCI.

EXERCISE 11.11

At the end of this exercise, you should be able to describe local customs and practices during pregnancy, childbirth, lactation and child feeding practices. **(CM 10.3)**

Mid-year population of a PHC in the year 2019 was 32,100. During the same year, 3700 children were born, and six maternal deaths were reported. A total of 310 infants died in 2019 among which 148 died after 28 days of their life. The medical officer was asked to report the following to the district health officials.

- Crude birth rate (CBR)
- Infant mortality rate (IMR)
- Maternal mortality ratio (MMR)
- Neonatal mortality rate (NMR), and
- Post neonatal mortality rate (PMR).

Guide Notes

- Indices of mortality and morbidity in under-5 children
- Steps under IMNCI.

EXERCISE 11.12

At the end of this exercise you should be able to enumerate and describe the methods of screening high risk groups and common health problems. **(CM 10.2)**

Devaki, a 17-year-old female, lives in a remote village of Bihar. She resides in a kuccha house with her husband and in-laws. Currently, she is pregnant and nearing full-term. She used to work as a daily wage labourer till the 8th month of her pregnancy. She used to have two meals a day. Her pregnancy is registered at the nearest health sub-centre although her ANC visits were irregular. She developed labor pain and was taken to the sub-centre. At the sub-centre, ANM assessed Devaki and she noticed difficulty in progression of her labor. She referred her to the nearest CHC for further management. But due to difficulty in availability of transport vehicle she reached CHC after 4 hours. At the CHC, assisted delivery was performed and she delivered a baby girl weighing 2300 g immediately after birth, it was found that the baby's heart rate is 90 bpm, her breathing is irregular and respiratory rate is decreased, muscles flaccid and reflexes absent. Her body colour is pink but extremities were blue.

- What is your assessment about the condition of the baby?
- What action should be taken after assessing the baby?
- What could have been done to prevent this condition?

Guide Notes

- Essential and emergency obstetrics care (EmOC)
- IYCF

- NSSK, JSSK, JSY, BFHI
- RMNCH+A, RMNCAH+N
- Steps under IMNCI.

EXERCISE 11.13

At the end of this exercise you should be able to enumerate and describe the methods of screening high risk groups and common health problems. **(CM 10.2)**

Sukanya is a 26-year-old pregnant female residing in a semi-urban area of Nalanda, Bihar. She lives in a pucca house with her husband and her mother. She is a housewife, and her husband is a farmer. Soon after detection of pregnancy, she was registered in the nearest health subcentre with the help of an ASHA. She attended all ANC check-ups and followed the advice. After the onset of labor pain, she rushed to the PHC. Her hemoglobin level at that time was found as 10.4 g/dl. After few hours, she delivered a male baby weighing 2700 g. At the time of birth, the baby's heart rate was 110 bpm, respiration was slow and irregular, he showed some flexion of extremities, grimace, and his body colour was pink but the extremities were blue. The child was resuscitated at the newborn care corner. At 5-minutes, the heart rate of the baby was 114 bpm, he was crying good, showed active movements in all the limbs, cried on checking reflex, but still the body was pink with blue extremities.

Calculate APGAR scores at 1-minute and 5-minute.

Guide Notes

- APGAR score
- Essential and emergency obstetrics care (EmOC)
- NSSK, JSSK, JSY, BFHI.

EXERCISE 11.14

At the end of this exercise you should be able to describe the reproductive, maternal, newborn and child health (RMCH); child survival and safe motherhood interventions. **(CM10.4)**

You are the Medical Officer in a PHC covering a population of 26,300. Birth rate of that area was reported to be 18/1000 populations in 2017. The labor room is available with facilities for conducting normal delivery. However, you are concerned about the number of deliveries taking place at that PHC. Reported institutional deliveries in that year were 206. Upon enquiring about the mode of delivery of pregnant females in your area, you find out that most of the pregnant females' did not register at the HSC and prefer home delivery. ASHAs and ANMs were also not conducting adequate visits to the houses of these pregnant females. Moreover, it was also found that home delivery was being conducted by untrained *dais*.

- Calculate the expected number of pregnancies per year in your PHC.
- What action(s) will you take to encourage institutional deliveries among pregnant women in your area?

Guide Notes

- ANC services provided at HSC, PHC, CHC, DH, tertiary hospitals
- Expected ANC cases in a community

- Role of ASHA, ANM, MHW
- Skilled and traditional birth attendants.

EXERCISE 11.15

At the end of this exercise you should be able to describe the reproductive, maternal, newborn and child health (RMCH); child survival and safe motherhood interventions. **(CM10.4)**

MBBS students of a medical college were taken to a health sub-centre (HSC) for an academic visit. At the HSC, they were explained about the facilities present there and their population coverage. The ANM told them that pregnant females from a particular village are reluctant for ANC check-ups and institutional delivery. The medical students were assigned a task to enquire about the reasons for the same. After visiting the village, they found that connectivity between village and the HSC is not an issue as pucca roads was present and the village was located within 5 km of the HSC. They inferred that the problem is mainly social, mostly related to unawareness. For conducting home deliveries, a local *dai* was available but she did not receive any formal training. It was also found that the measures of cleanliness were not being followed at the time of delivery. MBBS students were asked to:

- Suggest actions that were needed on a priority basis
- Enumerate the key messages to increase awareness about the importance of institutional delivery in the community.

Guide Notes

- Steps by government to encourage institutional delivery
- Skilled and Traditional birth attendants.

EXERCISE 11.16

At the end of this exercise you should be able to describe the reproductive, maternal, newborn and child health (RMCH); child survival and safe motherhood interventions. **(CM10.4)**

Rekha 27-year-old female, delivered a male baby at her home which is located in a village. On the 8th postpartum day, she developed fever, pain, and tenderness in her lower abdomen. She was taken to the nearest CHC for treatment. On detailed enquiry, it was found that after home delivery by a local *dai*, she was kept in a separate room with poor ventilation and inadequate natural light. The room and the bed were also not cleaned regularly. Instead of sterile sanitary napkins, she was using clothes for her lochial discharge. Till date, the ASHA made only one home visit to investigate the condition of the mother and her child.

- What is your probable diagnosis?
- What is the role of an ASHA regarding postnatal care in such cases?
- What suggestions should be given to the family members in such a condition?

Guide Notes

- IYCF
- NSSK, BFHI
- Role of ASHA, ANM, MHW
- WHO guideline for ANC and PNC visits.

EXERCISE 11.17

At the end of this exercise you should be able to enumerate and describe the methods of screening high risk groups and common health problems. **(CM 10.2)**

You are an undergraduate medical student and were allotted a family in the village during community medicine posting. The family allotted to you is a joint family comprising of seven members, including one 4-month pregnant female. This is her second pregnancy, and she delivered her last child one year ago. She was registered at the nearest HSC and availed her first ANC checkup. While examining her first ANC report, you noticed that her Hb level was 9.5 g/dl at that time. On further investigation, you find out that she is doing manual labour work intermittently, apart from taking care of all the household activities. Regarding her dietary intake, you observe that her protein and calorie intakes are inadequate, and she was also not taking iron and folic acid supplementation.

- Classify the severity of anemia in this pregnant woman
- What advice will you give her regarding anemia management?
- What messages would you confer to her family members?

Guide Notes

- Direct and indirect causes of maternal mortality
- Essential and Emergency obstetrics care (EmOC).

EXERCISE 11.18

At the end of this exercise you should be able to enumerate and describe the methods of screening high risk groups and common health problems. **(CM 10.2)**

Namita is a 24-year aged primigravida living in a periurban area, in a semi pucca house with her family. She is currently 8 months pregnant and registered at her nearest urban PHC for her ANC check-ups. One day when she presented for her ANC check-ups at the PHC, she expressed her unawareness and apprehension regarding breastfeeding practices after childbirth. As a medical officer of that urban PHC,

- Counsel her regarding practices to achieve safe and adequate breastfeeding, including the benefits of breastfeeding and breast milk, for the mother and the baby respectively
- Till what age, will you recommend her to breastfeed her baby?

Guide Notes

- IYCF
- BFHI.

EXERCISE 11.19

At the end of this exercise you should be able to describe the reproductive, maternal, newborn and child health (RMCH); child survival and safe motherhood interventions. **(CM 10.4)**

Jyotsana is a 22-year-old female belonging to a rural area of Bihar. She has a 4-month female child, currently on exclusive breastfeeding (EBF). However, she is worried and feels that her baby is not gaining enough weight. Moreover, she was also uncertain whether her breast milk alone is sufficient for the baby and wanted to introduce formula milk and other commercial food items to her child's feed. Her baby's birth weight was 2800 g, while current weight is 5800 g. Keeping these problems in mind, she visited the nearest PHC to consult a doctor.

- As a medical officer, what advice will you give regarding weight gain in her child?
- What advice regarding feeding the child, should be given to her?
- What are the signs of adequate breastfeeding, which you would want to educate her about?

Guide Notes

- EBF
- Supplementary food introduction and weaning off
- IYCF.

EXERCISE 11.20

At the end of this exercise you should be able to enumerate and describe the methods of screening high risk groups and common health problems. **(CM10.2)**

An evaluation of newborn and child health services was done across the state of Jharkhand. After completion of the evaluation, two districts were found to have unsatisfactory newborn and child health service delivery systems. Those two districts were having inadequate infrastructure and poorly trained or even untrained manpower to provide the fore mentioned healthcare services. Being a Chief Medical Officer (CMO) of one of two districts, you were directed to improve the existing health care delivery system for child health. You arranged a training session for medical and paramedical staffs on newborn and child health.

- What key messages will you confer regarding essential newborn care?
- How do you plan to improve the facilities for newborn care at each level of existing health care delivery system in these districts?

Guide Notes

- RMNCH+A, RMNCAH+N
- Screening tools used by frontline workers for screening of developmental defects in school going children
- Steps under IMNCI.

EXERCISE 11.21

At the end of this exercise you should be able to describe the physiology, clinical management and principles of adolescent health including ARSH. **(CM10.8)**

An adolescent girl comes to a PHC, with complaints of increased blood loss during menstruation (menorrhagia), weakness and abdominal pain during her menses. On inquiring you come to know that most girls in her friend circle are using unsanitary napkins. They were unaware of where to procure sanitary napkins from and the importance of using the same. As a medical officer of that centre, advise the girl regarding the points given below.

- Types of services and programs, under the government, which she can avail including their benefits
- Different sources for procuring economic and cheaper sanitary napkins
- Nutrition related and sexual health related education.

Guide Notes

- Adolescent friendly health services
- Global strategy for women's, children's, and adolescents' health
- Syndromic management of STDs/STIs.

REFERENCES

1. Kadri's IAPSM's textbook of Community Medicine. 2nd edn, pages 591–592, 602–603, 609, 614–616, 618, 626, 630–632, 636.
2. Park's Textbook of Preventive and Social Medicine. 26th edn, Chapter 11 'Preventive Medicine in Obstetrics, Pediatrics and Geriatrics' (602–682).

FURTHER READING

1. Chhabra P. Maternal Health. In: Kadri AM, editor. IAPSM's Textbook of Community Medicine. New Delhi: Jaypee; 2019. pp. 722–35.
2. Goyal P, Singh M, Lukhmana S. Reproductive Health, and Family Welfare. In: Kadri AM, editor.
3. Kaur R, Goel A D. Child Health. In: Kadri AM, editor. IAPSM's Textbook of Community Medicine. New Delhi: Jaypee; 2019. pp. 736–756.
4. Park K. Park's textbook of Preventive and Social Medicine. 25th ed. Jabalpur: Banarsidas Bhanot; 2019. pp. 590–93, 538–40, 576–81, 584–86, 610–30, 626–30, 616–18, 531–71.

CHAPTER 12

Family Planning

Competency code	Competency addressed	Exercise
CM9.4	Enumerate and describe the causes and consequences of population explosion and population dynamics of India.	12.8, 12.12
CM9.5	Describe the methods of population control	12.5, 12.7
CM9.6	Describe the National Population Policy	12.6
CM10.6	Enumerate and describe various family planning methods, their advantages and shortcomings	12.9, 12.10
CM10.7	Enumerate and describe the basis and principles of the Family Welfare Program including the organization, technical and operational aspects	12.3, 12.11
OG21.1	Describe and discuss the temporary and permanent methods of contraception, indications, technique and complications; selection of patients, side effects and failure rate including oral contraceptives (OCs), male contraception, emergency contraception and IUCD	12.1, 12.2, 12.4

EXERCISE 12.1

At the end of this exercise you should be able to describe and discuss the temporary and permanent methods of contraception, indications, technique and complications; selection of patients, side effects and failure rate including oral contraceptives (OCs), male contraception, emergency contraception and IUCD. **(OG21.1)**

Malti, a 24-years-old female, married for 1.5 years, delivered a female child 4 weeks ago. She was visited by an ASHA worker of the village. During this visit, Malti's mother-in-law told the ASHA worker about their preference for male child and insisted that Malti should conceive again soon. But Malti, who is a graduate, wants to space her next pregnancy by at least 3 years and wants to use contraceptive method. ASHA worker asked Malti and her mother-in-law to come for health education session scheduled after few days in the nearby health facility.

- What is 'contraceptive' and explain spacing methods and permanent methods of contraception?
- Which contraceptive choices would you suggest for Malti?
- Which health promotion strategy could be helpful in given condition introduced under 'Mission Parivar Vikas'.

- Enumerate the provisions stated under MTP act for terminating any pregnancy?
- What are the amendments in 'The Medical Termination of Pregnancy (Amendment) Act, 2020'?

Guide Notes

- MTP Act 1972
- Amendments in MTP Act (2020).

EXERCISE 12.7

At the end of this exercise you should be able to describe the methods of population control. **(CM9.5)**

Rohit, a 36-year, medical representative, is a father of 2 children among which, the younger one is 5-years-old. He visits the OPD and tells his doctor that his family is complete and wants to adopt some terminal method of contraception. His wife is hypertensive and had 2 caesarean sections and is unwilling to undergo any surgical procedure, so they have decided to go for vasectomy. But he is afraid that this procedure might affect his potency and libido (as told by his colleagues).

- How would you counsel the patient regarding his concerns?
- What are permanent or irreversible methods of family planning (FP)?

Guide Notes

- Permanent methods of family planning
- Under-trial male contraceptive pills.

EXERCISE 12.8

At the end of this exercise you should be able to enumerate and describe the causes and consequences of population explosion and population dynamics of India. **(CM9.4)**

A 21-year woman comes to your outpatient clinic for a visit. Upon entering the room, you see a well- nourished patient in no apparent distress. The patient introduces herself and gives no significant medical history. She informs that she recently relocated to Bengaluru from Mumbai where she worked in an advertising agency. She is in a live-in relationship and want to discuss options for birth control.

Then you ask her what she has used in the past for birth control. She reports that she has been taking birth control pills (BCPs) for the past two years, but she often forgets to take her pills daily.

Her social history includes a distant history of smoking and currently one sexual partner. Two years ago, she was diagnosed with *Chlamydia* and was treated with antibiotics. Her STD was diagnosed at a hospital after that her then boyfriend developed symptoms. She has never had pelvic inflammatory disease (PID) and re-tested negative for STDs a year ago after breaking up with her boyfriend. On asking whether she has been using birth control pills for contraception or any other medical problems, such as endometriosis, she informs that she has had two previous sexual relationships with men and was using birth control for contraception. She was also concurrently using condoms to prevent STDs. She denies any previous pregnancies, miscarriages, or live births. She did not experience any side-effects from her birth control pills. However, she was not taking her birth control pills consistently.

- What are contraceptive choices for a nulliparous female in this case scenario?
- What is Pearl's Index?

Guide Notes

- Advantages and disadvantages of different types of contraceptives
- Failure rate of contraceptives and Pearl index.

EXERCISE 12.9

At the end of this exercise you should be able to enumerate and describe various family planning methods, their advantages and shortcomings. **(CM 10.6)**

A second year PG student of Department of Respiratory Medicine, experienced myalgia with fever, during her ward visits. She reported to her consultant that for the last few days she is experiencing weakness, evening rise of temperature and her morning sputum was slightly blood tinged. She has also had productive cough for the last 15 days. Because of her busy schedule she was ignoring the symptoms but today she was not able to get up for her ward rounds and hence came to see him. She is 28-year-old, married for 2 years and had her last menstrual period (LMP) 10 days back. After extensive investigations and clinical examinations, she was diagnosed positive for 'tuberculosis' and under 'newly diagnosed category', appropriate regimen was started as per RNTCP guidelines. Considering her condition, her unit head granted her a leave of 15 days.

She reported back to the institute and joined her duties. After 2 months of coming back she started feeling nauseated in the morning. She also noticed that she missed her menstrual period too. She consulted obstetrician for that matter. On history taking, they found that she was regularly taking oral contraceptive pills (OCPs) for the last 2 years and no history of missed pills was there. On examination, pallor, icterus, oedema was absent, but Hegar's sign was positive. Her routine investigations were done along with urine pregnancy test (UPT). All her reports were under normal range and UPT was positive.

- What was the reason of contraceptive failure in this case?
- While prescribing medication for treatment of tuberculosis, what are the important points to be considered for counselling of the subject?
- Discuss contraceptive choices for the females who are taking 'enzymatic inhibitors' for any other ailment.

Guide Notes

- Contraception failure
- Enzymatic inhibitors and activators.

EXERCISE 12.10

At the end of this exercise you should be able to enumerate and describe various family planning methods, their advantages and shortcomings. **(CM 10.6)**

Reena, 24-year-old primigravida, delivered a healthy male baby, 3.5 months back, by caesarean section at 36 weeks of gestation due to foetal distress. She stayed in hospital for 5 days and was counselled for nutrition, breastfeeding, and contraceptive measures. Reena decides to rely on lactational amenorrhea as a method of contraception. During her visit to hospital for vaccination of her child at 14 weeks, she met her doctor with the complaint of generalized weakness. She has not regained menstrual cycle and is not using any contraceptive after last delivery. After the examination, doctor asked Reena to take UPT, which came positive. On history taking, she informed that the child was top fed due to inadequate milk production and poor latching of the child. She also reported that they never used any contraceptive as she assumed that she could not conceive so soon after delivery.

- What could be the cause of accidental pregnancy in this case.
- What are the causes of failure of lactational amenorrhea as contraceptive measure?
- What is the failure rate of lactation amenorrhea method (LAM)?

Guide Notes

- Different types of natural methods of family planning (FP)
- 12 pillars of reproductive health
- Determinants of reproductive health at all stages of life.

EXERCISE 12.11

At the end of this exercise you should be able to enumerate and describe the basis and principles of the Family Welfare Program including the organization, technical and operational aspects. **(CM10.7)**

A young couple, woman aged 20 years and the man aged 24 years, married for 2 months, come to see the FP service provider. They were using condoms as the barrier method of contraception, but last night somehow during the sexual act, the condom broke, due to which they are afraid of a resultant pregnancy. They absolutely want to postpone their first child for at least one year until they both complete their studies. Now they do not want to rely only on condoms.

- What suggestions should be given by the healthcare provider to avoid pregnancy?
- What instructions should be given for use of emergency contraceptive pills (ECPs)?
- What will the service provider suggest regarding postponement of pregnancy?

Guide Note

- Emergency contraceptives.

EXERCISE 12.12

At the end of this exercise you should be able to enumerate and describe the causes and consequences of population explosion and population dynamics of India. **(CM9.4)**

A 26-year-old female, married for 5 years, mother of a 3-year-old child, came to the health facility with complaint of amenorrhea for 6 weeks, pain in the lower abdomen and spotting since morning. On asking about contraceptive history, she mentions that two years back she decided to go for IUCD insertion as her compliance for OCPs was poor and the couple wanted to have spacing. Her abdominal examination revealed tenderness in the lower region. On per speculum and per vaginal examination, no IUCD thread was found. Urine pregnancy test of the patient was positive and trans-abdominal ultra-sonography (TAS) confirmed missing IUCD and absence of any intrauterine sac. On trans-vaginal sonography (TVS) an ectopic pregnancy was located.

- What could be the reason of ectopic pregnancy?
- What are important points of counselling in IUCD users?
- What is a GATHER approach in counselling?

Guide Notes

- Side effects of IUDs
- GATHER approach in counselling.

REFERENCES

1. Kadri's IAPSM's Textbook of Community Medicine. 2nd Edition, pages 591, 592, 594, 602, 603, 604 (591–606).
2. PARK's Textbook of Preventive and Social Medicine. 26th edn, pages 572, 574, 586, 591.

FURTHER READING

1. MTP amendment bill 2020. Available from: http://164.100.47.4/BillsTexts/LSBillTexts/Asintroduced/55_2020_LS_Eng.pdf
2. OPCs and Antibiotics. Available from https://www.ncbi.nlm.nih.gov/pmc/articles/PMC3250726/#:~:text=Rifampin%20is%20the%20on ly%20antibiotic%20to%20date%20that%20has%20been,birth%20control%20while%

CHAPTER

13

Health System

Competency code	Competency addressed	Exercise
CM5.7	Describe food hygiene	13.6
CM10.4	Describe the reproductive, maternal, newborn and child health (RMCH); child survival and safe motherhood interventions	13.3
CM13.2 CM13.4	Describe disaster management cycle Describe the details of the National Disaster Management Authority	13.4
CM17.3 CM17.5	Describe primary health care, its components and principles Describe healthcare delivery in India	13.5
CM20.1	List important public health events of last five years	13.1
CT1.15	Prescribe an appropriate anti-tuberculosis regimen based on the location of disease, smear positivity and negativity and comorbidities based on current national guidelines including directly observed tuberculosis therapy (DOTS)	13.2

EXERCISE 13.1

At the end of this exercise, you should be able to list important public health events of last five years. **(CM20.1)**

A healthcare worker travelled from Darjeeling to Kolkata, in April 2020, and came back after a span of seven days. His return journey by road, along with 5 other health care workers, was uneventful owing to then ongoing national lockdown, which rendered roadways unpopulated. They were to stay in separate rooms in a big boarding hotel, where several other people from different professions were also temporarily residing. Three days later, one of the HCWs developed fever with sore throat, who thereafter tested positive for COVID-19 upon consulting the nearest government healthcare facility. The other co-passengers were informed about the report and were directed to get tested. They, however, went back to Kolkata the very next day by a private vehicle.

- What standard measures the health care workers should have followed?
- What major defaults are noted in handling of the case?
- Which necessary public health measure should have been implemented in this scenario?

Guide Note

- Guidelines for containment of COVID-19 suspects: Beginning v/s Now.

EXERCISE 13.2

At the end of this exercise, you should be able to prescribe an appropriate anti-tuberculosis regimen based on the location of disease, smear positivity and negativity and comorbidities based on current national guidelines including directly observed tuberculosis therapy (DOTS). **(CT1.15)**

A married nulliparous lady, aged 32-years, visited the nearest sub-centre for a regular health check-up as she is currently on ATT medications for Tuberculosis, which revealed that she is having BMI value on the underweight side. She has been married for three years and is yet to conceive. Upon enquiring, she told the doctor that she lives with her in-laws who prefer a grandson. She is concerned that she has infertility and bears the social brunt of it. On further probing it was made known that the husband was a truck driver. She was given her DOTS medication and sent home.

- Which medical and social problems exist in the above vignette?
- Advice preventive health practices to the lady in the above scenario.
- Explain the role of a public health activist here in this situation.

Guide Notes

- HRGs, at-risk population, bridge population.
- HSS plus.

EXERCISE 13.3

At the end of this exercise, you should be able to describe the reproductive, maternal, newborn and child health (RMCH); child survival and safe motherhood interventions. **(CM10.4)**

Harsh climates are witnessed in Darjeeling during winters. On one chilly night, in a hilly area of Kalimpong, Sheetal started having labor pains. Despite prior intimation to the nearest sub-centre, the ANM could not be contacted due to intense fog and cold. The family was dependent on the ANM's instructions till the last minute and hence did not know how to reach an FRU though there was one nearby. The child was delivered at home by Sheetal's untrained mother-in-law. Sheetal suffered postpartum hemorrhage (PPH) and died within 3days of the delivery. On the fourth day, the child perished to neonatal tetanus. Unfortunately, such situations are yet prevalent in such hilly terrains.

- What primary concern should have been addressed beforehand to prevent such incidences?
- Enlist the failures in the public health system which can be strengthened? And how?
- What is BPCR and how could it be followed here?

Guide Note

- Birth preparedness and complication readiness (BPCR) interventions.

EXERCISE 13.4

- At the end of this exercise, you should be able to describe disaster management cycle. **(CM13.2)**
- Describe the details of the National Disaster Management Authority. **(CM13.4)**

An earthquake was reported in a tea garden area dominated primarily by its tribal population. Its occurrence was anticipated as there had been foreshocks. Soon after it was followed by floods, which further hampered the already crumbled water supply of the area. The resulting picture was a huge catastrophe, with death tolls continually

CHAPTER

14

Health Management

Competency code	Competency addressed	Exercise
CM8.2	Describe and discuss the epidemiological and control measures including the use of essential laboratory tests at the primary care level for non-communicable diseases (diabetes, hypertension, stroke, obesity and cancer, etc.)	14.9
CM11.3	Enumerate and describe specific occupational health hazards, their risk factors and preventive measures	14.10
CM16.3	Describe health management techniques.	14.1, 14.3, 14.5–14.8, 14.10–14.14
CM16.4	Describe health planning in India and National policies related to health and health planning	14.4
CM17.5	Describe healthcare delivery in India	14.2, 14.4
CM20.3	Describe any event important to health of the community	14.11
MI8.16	Describe the National Health Programs in the prevention of common infectious disease (for information purpose only as taught in CM).	
PH1.55	Describe and discuss the following National Health programs including immunization, tuberculosis, leprosy, malaria, HIV, filaria, kala azar, diarrheal diseases, anemia and nutritional disorders, blindness, non-communicable diseases, cancer and iodine deficiency.	14.1

HUMAN RESOURCE MANAGEMENT

EXERCISE 14.1

- At the end of the exercise, you should be able to describe Health management techniques. **(CM16.3)**
- Describe and discuss the following National Health Programs including immunization, tuberculosis, leprosy, malaria, HIV, filaria, kala azar, diarrheal diseases, anemia and nutritional disorders, blindness, non-communicable diseases, cancer and iodine deficiency. **(PH1.55)**
- Describe the National Health Programs in the prevention of common infectious disease (for information purpose only as taught in CM). **(MI8.16)**

In this exercise, you would first identify a healthcare delivery system (either a healthcare facility or a health programme) under supervision of a facilitator / mentor. Once the name of the facility is decided, identify the organizational structure of the healthcare delivery system.

Suggested options are:

- Government healthcare facility
  - Primary health centre (PHC)
  - Community health centre (CHC)
  - District hospital (DH)
  - Public funded medical college
- Private healthcare facility
  - Not-for-profit trust or NGO hospital
  - For-profit private clinic or primary/secondary level hospital
  - For-profit private tertiary level non-academic hospital
  - For-profit private tertiary academic hospital
- Health programme
  - National Health Mission
  - National Tuberculosis Elimination Programme (previously Tuberculosis Control Programme or RNTCP)
  - National Vector Borne Disease Control Programme (NVBDCP)
  - National Programme for Prevention and Control of Cancers, Diabetes, Cardio-vascular Diseases and Stroke (NPCDCS)
  - National Programme for Healthcare of Elderly (NPHCE)

Develop an organogram for the chosen health facility or programme with names, designations and hierarchical place of people working there.

EXERCISE 14.2

At the end of the exercise, you should be able to describe healthcare delivery in India. **(CM17.5)**

- Develop a time-motion job analysis plan (direct observation or work diary) for the job of ASHA. Conduct the time-motion job analysis using your plan.
- Develop a job model for an ASHA depending on the information obtained in exercise
- You can use the draft job model provided in **Fig. 14.1** by a research team.

Guide Notes

- Eligibility and recruitment of ASHA
- Roles and responsibilities of ASHA.

EXERCISE 14.3

At the end of the exercise, you should be able to describe health management techniques. **(CM16.3)**

Make a table to show the human resource mapping for a designated health facility (e.g., PHC/CHC/DH) or a programme (e.g., NHM/NTEP/NVBDCP/NPCDCS/NPHCE etc.). An example for such a mapping of NPCDCS at district level is given in **Table 14.1**.

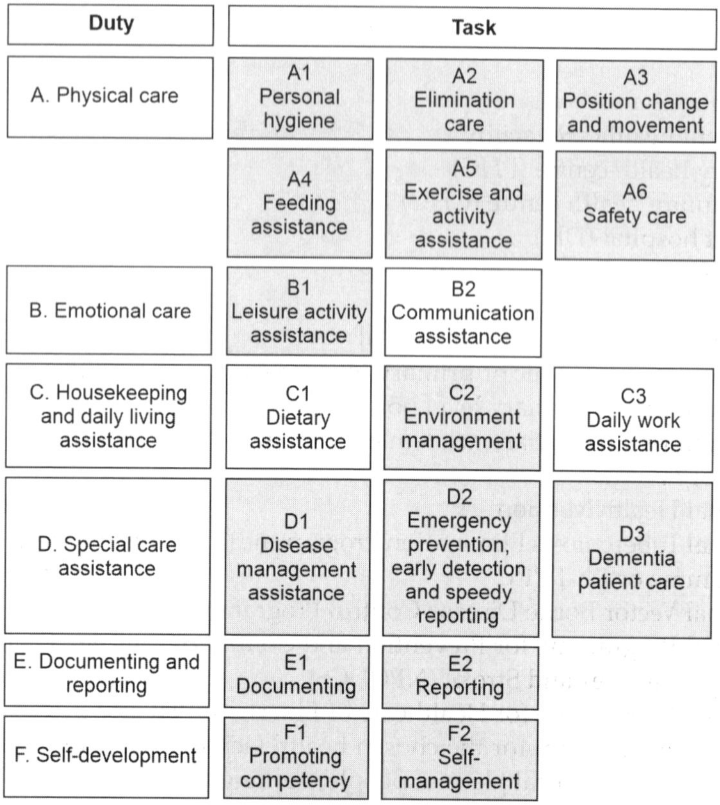

Fig. 14.1: Job model of care.

TABLE 14.1: NPCDCS Human Resource Mapping (District/ State)

Sr. No.	*Designation of Human Resource*	*Type*	*Sanctioned*	*In Place*	*Balance (Deficit/ Excess)*
1.	District Programme Manager	Core			
2.	District Programme Coordinator	Core			
3.	Finance-cum-Logistics Coordinator	Core			
4.	Data Entry Operator	Core			
5.	Cardiologist	Shared			
6.	Oncologist	Shared			
7.	Pathologist	Shared			
8.	Ophthalmologist	Shared			
9.	Gynecologist	Shared			
10.	Surgeon	Shared			
11.	Dental Surgeon	Shared			
12.	Physician	Shared			
13.	Medical Officer (Male)	Shared			
14.	Medical Officer (Female)	Shared			

Contd...

Contd...

Sr. No.	Designation of Human Resource	Type	Sanctioned	In Place	Balance (Deficit/ Excess)
15.	Staff Nurses	Shared			
16.	Laboratory Technician	Shared			
17.	Physiotherapist	Shared			
18.	Counsellor	Core			
19.	ANM/ Health Worker	Shared			
20.	ASHA	Shared			
21.	Anganwadi Worker	Shared			

- Four posts for staff nurses in a district hospital of Odisha are vacant. The process of recruitment needs to be started for these posts.
  - Establish the recruitment rules.
  - Draft an advertisement to be placed in various newspapers.
  - Develop the application form which the participants can either fill online or download from the website and submit via offline mode.

Guide Notes

- NPCDCS and NMAP
  In continuation with above exercise, after posting the advertisement, more than 200 application forms have been received till the last date of submission. Due to the large number of applications, the administration wants to screen the applicants for eligibility before conducting a recruitment test
- Develop a screening format which would be used for this purpose by the document verification committee
  Continuing with the recruitment process of the staff nurses, screening of application forms is over now. The number of candidates eligible to undergo the selection process after this screening is158. The candidates need to go through a double-stepped selection process in the form of a written test, followed by an interviewing-person. These 158 eligible candidates would appear for the written test after 4 weeks and for the interview 6 weeks after the written test
- Develop a set of 20 multiple choice questions (MCQs) or extended matching questions (EMQs) for the written test
- Develop a question bank of 50 short answer type questions for the interview
- Steps in scientific planning
- Health planning
  The processes of written test and interview are over now. The successful candidates would be sent an appointment letter with instructions which are to be followed during reporting for joining the job
- Draft an appointment letter for the staff nurses, successfully passing the recruitment procedure, who can now join the posts.

TRAINING NEED ASSESSMENT

EXERCISE 14.4

- At the end of the exercise, you should be able to describe health planning in India and National policies related to health and health planning. **(CM16.4)**
- Describe healthcare delivery in India. **(CM17.5)**

The PGs need to conduct training need assessment (TNA) of any cadre of workers (preferably frontline field workers) in any one domain of their work profile and present it in the department. This activity is designed to make the students learn about the process of TNA, and to identify and differentiate training and non-training needs of the workers.

The students must work under the following broad guidelines to assess the training needs:

- Health system goals with regards to a particular health problem of concern
- Identify the role of the health worker in accomplishing that goal
- Identify the training domains (knowledge, skill, emotions, etc.) that health workers require, to perform the job effectively
- Identify the discrepancies or gaps between an employee's skills and the skills required by them for effective performance at their current job, through qualitative and quantitative data collection methods
- Plan and present the findings
- Submit a report and plan a training program for concerned cadre of workers. (It is preferable to conduct this assessment for field level workers.)

Assessment Format for TNA

Sr. No.	*Parameter*	*Marks (5 each)*
1.	Rationale for selection of cadre of healthcare personnel	
2.	Method used to assess training needs	
3.	Data analysis and presentation	
4.	Implementation of training	
5.	Training evaluation plan	
6.	Conducting evaluation of training	

Guide Notes

- Training need assessment (TNA).

PLANNING THE TRAINING

EXERCISE 14.5

At the end of the exercise, you should be able to describe health management techniques. **(CM16.3)**

You are the MO at a PHC in Lutera Khurd (Punjab). You have received an order from CMHO regarding upgradation of all the sub-centre in your area to health and wellness centers (HWCs) from the upcoming year. Accordingly, the whole staff of these health sub-centre need to be trained. Out of the 12 training packages provided under HWC guidelines, the first seven packages would be initiated with immediate effect, through these HWCs. The training can be provided either at the DH or the PHC itself. The trainers for first three batches would be master trainers from state and district levels. Afterwards, the district programme managers or CHC BMOs, if required, will be conducting the trainings.

- Make a training need summary for the HWC training of your staff.

Category of staff to be trained	*Duration of training*	*Venue*	*Batch size*	*Total training load*			*Target no of batches for next year*
				Sanctioned strength	In position	Total untrained load	

- Based on the summary, develop the anticipated budget proposal for the annual training under HWC domain in a tabular format (a draft is given in **Table 14.2**).

TABLE 14.2: Draft budget for 3 days training programme of medical officers andstaff nurses in NCDs under NPCDCS

Sr. No.	*Budget head*	*Unit cost*	*Units*	*Total cost*	*Remark*
1	Training Faculty				
1.1	Honorarium for faculty (per session)	1500	12	18000	The honorarium would be given to faculty trainers that would be Rs. 1500/session. Each session would be of 45 minutes (minimum).
2	Participants (MOs/SNs)				
2.1	Accommodation for participants	2000	30	60000	Accommodation needs to be provided for 25–30 persons for 2 days. Room rate is expected to be Rs. 2000/day on twin sharing basis. Fifteen rooms would be required every day.
2.2	Vehicle hiring for local movement of participants	4000	3	12000	One 30 seated vehicle would be needed for movement of participants from place of accommodation to training venue.
2.3	Meals for participants	350	100	35000	The meals include lunch (Rs. 250) and tea/snacks twice (Rs. 100) for 30 participants and 5–10 faculty members for 3 days.
3	Training kit	1500	30	45000	Twenty-five kits for participants and five kits for faculty would be prepared. Participant's kit will include one training module and stationary items such as bag/folder, notebook, pen, pencil, pen-drive etc. Faculty's kit will have a facilitator module apart from other stationary items.
4	Venue charges	3000	3	9000	Charge of using Board Room has been set as Rs. 3000/day by competent authority.
5	Human resources				
5.1	Two multipurpose assistant (on daily basis)	400	6	2400	The Multipurpose Assistant would help in all the petty works during training days.
5.2	One training coordinator (for 7 days)	1500	7	10500	The training coordinator would take care of all communications, record maintenance, reporting and facilitate the day-to-day activities during the training. She/he would be hired for 7 days (2 days before + 3 days during + 2 days after the training) to facilitate the process.
6	Contingency/ overheads (@5%)			9595	Overhead charges for the institute would be covered through this. Cost of accounting and audit by the empanelled auditor of institute and other unforeseen expenses would also be covered through this.
	Total			201495	

2. Now classify these task according to their urgency and/or importance in respective cells (four categories) of the table below.

	Urgent	*Not Urgent*
Important		
Not Important		

3. Which of these tasks can and should be shifted from their cell with reason?

SUPERVISION AND MONITORING

As a manager, you need to supervise your staff periodically to identify any bottlenecks in performance, outputs, and outcomes.

EXERCISE 14.9

At the end of the exercise, you should be able describe and discuss the epidemiological and control measures including the use of essential laboratory tests at the primary care level for non-communicable diseases (diabetes, hypertension, stroke, obesity and cancer, etc.) **(CM 8.2)**

Various programs in our healthcare system have nodal officers either at state or district level. One of their functions is to periodically supervise their subordinates. For example, in the NPCDCS the NCD state nodal officers must visit the 'NCD Clinics' and 'NCD cells' at district level.

- Develop a supervisory visit checklist which can be used by NCD state nodal officer during visits to the NCD clinics and district NCD cells (use the NCD action plan to identify the facility or district level targets/indicators)
- Use the given supervisory visit checklist to assess the performance of an assigned health facility.

Guide Notes

- NCD clinics and NCD cells
- NITI Aayog
- Three-year action agenda of Niti Aayog.

JOB SATISFACTION AND MOTIVATION

EXERCISE 14.10

- At the end of the exercise you should be able to enumerate and describe specific occupational health hazards, their risk factors and preventive measures. **(CM 11.3)**
- Describe health management techniques. **(CM 16.3)**

Despite providing adequate training and remuneration (salary, other allowances etc.), some of the staff members were found to be only suboptimally functional. It was reported that they are not satisfied with their jobs.

You would be given names of such human resource personnel(s) for assessment of job satisfaction and motivation. You need to conduct interviews with this/these personnel(s) to determine the level of job satisfaction they have, the factors which affect satisfaction and motivation etc. Before conducting these interviews, you should read Maslow' hierarchy of need theory and understand the model (five levels of needs: Physiological, safety and security, social, self-esteem and self-actualization).

- Make a list of factors which the personnel(s) consider important for satisfaction with job and motivation for day-to-day activities as well as long-time performance
- Now categorize these factors into one of the five groups of motivators, accordingly in the table given below. Use a separate table for each personnel.

Sr. No.	Motivator	Factors expressed by the personnel(s)
1.	Physiological needs	
2.	Safety and security needs	
3.	Social needs	
4.	Self-esteem needs	
5.	Self-actualization needs	

- Now use the list of motivating factors developed in 'Part 2' of this exercise. Ask the employee to rank these motivating factors, with number '1' being the most important motivator. More than one motivator may share a common rank.

Sr. No.	Motivating factors	Rank
1.		
2.		
3.		
4.		

Guide Note

- Maslow' Hierarchy of need theory.

CONFLICT MANAGEMENT

EXERCISE 14.11

- At the end of the exercise, you should be able to describe health management techniques. **(CM16.3)**
- Describe any event important to health of the community. **(CM 20.3)**

Recall a recent situation in your workplace where your responsibility as a leader was to manage the conflict. Complete the following 'Conflict Identification and Description' exercise. Complete all the rows of the table given below.

Sr. No.	Steps	Response
1.	*Conflict situation:* Describe the situation of conflict from the scenario	
2.	What you did? (Write evaluative statements about your approach)	
3.	Consequences (Describe the effects of your approach)	
4.	Feelings (Describe your negative/positive feelings)	
5.	What could have been done otherwise? (Write statements disputing your approach)	
6.	New feelings (positive/negative)	

Different types of managers and health system leaders use their own conflict management methods. Conduct interviews with five managers/senior persons from different levels of health system. Inform them that you would be recording these interviews for your training exercise. In the interviews, ask them to recollect one or more instances of conflict and how they managed those. Also ask them about the measures they have taken in the organization for conflict management in the future.

- After the interview, show them the following table and ask what rank they give to the following conflict management methods. Use separate table for each manager/senior person.

Sr. No.	Resolution approach	Rank for conflict management
1.	Preventing conflict	
2.	Suppressing the conflict	
3.	Avoiding the conflict	
4.	Laughing at the conflict (Using false emotions for distracting the conflict)	
5.	Eliminating the conflict	
6.	Accepting the conflict	
7.	Recognizing the value of conflict	
8.	Encouraging the interpersonal criticism	
9.	Enhancing the conflict	
10.	Inducing the conflict	
11.	Managing the conflict	

- Once you have finished the interviews, you need to transcribe all those interviews. Now, read these transcripts and decide what is the rank for conflict management which you think these managers/senior persons give for conflict management (based on actual conflict examples they discussed)

Sr. No.	Resolution approach	Type of manager (designation)	Rank for conflict management
1.	Preventing conflict		
2.	Suppressing the conflict		
3.	Avoiding the conflict		
4.	Laughing at the conflict (using false emotions for distracting the conflict)		
5.	Eliminating the conflict		
6.	Accepting the conflict		
7.	Recognizing the value of conflict		
8.	Encouraging the interpersonal criticism		
9.	Enhancing the conflict		
10.	Inducing the conflict		
11.	Managing the conflict		

In a CHC, a staff nurse was posted for NPCDCS (NCD clinic staff nurse). NCD clinic staff nurse is trained in NCD clinic related services. In the CHC, all the staff nurses work in a well-coordinated manner. Every three months, the NCD clinic staff nurse must do a night duty for seven consecutive days, under RCH services, as per the roster. This results in the unavailability of trained staff nurse for NCD during that entire week.

- Is there a human resource conflict situation here?
- What type of conflict has been depicted in the above scenario?
- How would you solve this conflict?

Read the following report on conflict event, which has been prepared by the inquiry team.

Venue of conflict: Meeting Hall of CMHO's office

Date and time: 3rd July 2020, 12:50 pm

On the day of the monthly meeting at CMHO's office in the district Bardhana, Dy. CMHO, BMOs and MOs from various CHCs and PHCs, a few specialists, district level programme managers, and development partner representatives were present.

Dr Ganesh Sikdar, a MO, had fixed up a prior appointment with the CMHO's PA in connection with discussing some issues. As he approached the meeting room, he saw a Dy. CMHO, Dr Dwivedi conversing with the PA. He waited for some time outside. As the time of the meeting was nearing, he went inside the PA's room to remind him of his appointment. Due to the interruption, Dr Dwivedi got agitated and shouted at Dr Sikdar, called him an idiot and asked him to leave the room. Dr Sikdar, tearfully, reported the matter to the other MOs, who got infuriated and took it as an insult to the whole group. Meanwhile, other members of the group, the district programme managers, and other specialists, also started flocking around Dr Sikdar to find out what had happened. After knowing the details, they advised Dr Sikdar to forget about the incident and seek a fresh appointment with the PA. At this, a strong reaction came from the MOs resulting into big shouts, abuses, heated arguments and even some physical attacks. Suddenly two groups, apparently District Hospital and Periphery were formed, comprising of doctors working at the District Hospital and MOs working in the periphery. Slogans like "We want justice, and we want respect" could be heard from MOs' side. The CMHO came out of his room after hearing the loud voices. He also heard loud statements like "You always harass and suppress the juniors and never acknowledge the work they do with such meagre resources". Hurriedly, one of the MOs briefed the CMHO about what had happened. After hearing, he called Dr Sikdar and some other MOs to his room. The group requested the CMHO for immediate justice in the form of a written apology from Dr Dwivedi. The CMHO then called Dr Dwivedi and a few of his group members inside to hear their version and informed them about the MOs' demand for written apology, to which Dr Dwivedi refused to abide.

At this point, the CMHO was wondering how to conduct the monthly meeting. He started thinking about ways to end the conflict. He decided to arrange a direct confrontation meeting between the two groups.

- What are the main issues here?
- Why are these issues important?
- Who is responsible for resolving the issue?
- What precisely are the objectives for resolution?
- What possible course of action is available?
- How realistic is each of the actions/solutions proposed?
- What are the possible consequences since Dr Dwivedi refused to apologize?

Guide Note

- Frustrations and conflicts.

SELF-APPRAISAL IN A TEAM

EXERCISE 14.12

At the end of the exercise you should be able to describe health management techniques. **(CM16.3)**

This exercise is to motivate the human resource personnel(s) to conduct self-appraisal with the intent to improve teamwork. You should refer to the section on 'Johari Window', which will be used during this exercise. In Johari Window, the personnel(s) who agree to participate and get self-evaluated vis-à-vis, the model should be ready to get them evaluated.

Instructions for Johari Window Exercise:

- Collect the list of adjectives of Johari Window Exercise from your facilitator.
- Identify the name of the staff member who has agreed to get himself/herself evaluated.
- Identify the co-workers of this staff member. At least 50% of the co-workers need to be identified and prepared to participate in this exercise.
- Share the list of adjectives with the staff member and his/her coworkers.
- The person receiving feedback will choose 12 adjectives that best describe them.
- The other participants will each choose 8 adjectives that best describe the individual receiving the feedback.
- Each participant will reveal one adjective, which they feel represents the individual being assessed. Ask the individual if the adjective was on their list. If yes, place it in the OPEN box and if it is not, place it in the BLIND BOX.
- Continue around the group one by one until there has been at least 10 OPEN adjectives listed.
- The individual is then asked to reveal any remaining adjective that has not yet been identified by the participating coworkers. It may be that an individual identified the adjective, but the sharing process ended before that adjective was revealed. If this happens add it to the OPEN box. If no one has an adjective that the individual reveals, then it should be placed in the BLIND box.
- After the documentation has been completed, the participants can be asked the following questions:
    - Which elements of this exercise were novice to you?
    - Which adjectives may be helpful to you since now you know others' perspectives and observations?
    - What hidden adjectives would you like to show more often to your team members? What would be the first step you could take to move in this direction?

Guide Note

- Johari window exercise.

PERFORMANCE APPRAISAL

EXERCISE 14.13

At the end of the exercise you should be able to describe health management techniques. **(CM16.3)**

Healthcare staff need to be evaluated periodically to identify their performance status and decide on rewards or penalties.

- Identify the performance appraisal mechanism in the government healthcare system at the level of district hospital.
- Use the format available for performance appraisal to discuss its usefulness with
  - A supervising staff
  - A subordinate staff

Guide Notes

- Steps of evaluation of health services
- Elements of evaluation.

LEADERSHIP STYLE

EXERCISE 14.14

At the end of the exercise you should be able to describe health management techniques. **(CM16.3)**

Dr Kishore Singh is an orthopedic specialist and is posted as a Civil Surgeon at Malhari, Bihar. He has been on this post for approximately 3 years. He is rated by many as one of the most efficient doctors with good administrative skills. He is considered an intelligent, tactful, and effective leader by all, including his superiors.

As part of his organizational duties, Dr Singh directs four units of his hospital through his competent management skills and aggressive executive influence. These units are named units A, B, C and D within the hospital, and are headed by Dr Saldana, Dr Varshney, Dr Jain and Dr Qureshi, respectively. All these four doctors, working with Dr Singh, adhere to his advice and guidance whenever received for the day-to-day functioning of their respective units.

During a particular week, Dr Singh went on an inspection of the four units under his control. First, he went to Unit A (Physiotherapy), which was under Dr Saldana. In this unit, the procedures and overall goals were well understood by the ones involved in carrying them out as well as the patients. During the round Dr Singh was informed that some of the tasks recommended for implementation of patient welfare had not yet been completed by the group. Dr Singh asked Dr Saldana to get the things done by giving some incentives to her subordinates, along with close monitoring of their performances. He asked Dr Saldana to keep him posted about any progress as and when achieved.

Dr Singh then went to Unit B (Psychiatry), which was under Dr Varshney. In this unit as well, the overall goals were well understood and supported. However, as the situation will have it, Dr Singh expected high quality work and service delivery from this unit. During questioning, he found that some of the allotted tasks had not been completed, and hence he became a little thoughtful. After some time, he advised Dr Varshney to focus on increasing coordination among his staff by paying a more attention to his interpersonal relationships with them through good communication and counselling.

Thereafter, he went on to inspect Unit C (ICU) and Unit D (Blood Bank), where the nature of work he perceived as challenging. Work life in these units was known to be tough and involved higher degrees of risk while decision taking to achieve the

Contd...

Competency code	Competency addressed	Exercise
PE17.1	State the vision and outline the goals, strategies and plan of action of NHM and other important national programs pertaining to maternal and child health including RMNCH A+, RBSK, RKSK, JSSK mission Indradhanush and ICDS	15.6, 15.7
PE18.3	Conduct antenatal examination of women independently and apply at-risk approach in antenatal care	15.14
PE19.1	Describe the age related nutritional needs of infants, children and adolescents including micronutrients and vitamins	15.4
PE19.3	Vaccine description with regard to classification of vaccines, strain used, dose, route, schedule, risks, benefits and side effects, indications and contraindications	15.12
PE34.4	Discuss the preventive strategies adopted and the objectives and outcome of the National Tuberculosis Control Program	15.2
PH1.55	Describe and discuss the following National Health programs including immunization, tuberculosis, leprosy, malaria, HIV, filaria, kala azar, diarrheal diseases, anemia and nutritional disorders, blindness, non-communicable diseases, cancer and iodine deficiency	15.13, 15.16
PY9.6	Enumerate the contraceptive methods for male and female. Discuss their advantages and disadvantages	15.18

EXERCISE 15.1

At the end of the exercise you should be able to describe national policies related to health and health planning and millennium development goals. **(CM 17.4)**

The dynamic and evolving healthcare system in India has resulted in a significant decline in the maternal mortality ratio (MMR) in the country from 254 per 1 lakh live births in 2004-06 to 122 per 1 lakh live birth in the year 2015–17. Health being a state subject in the country, assessing these health care indicators at state level or below provides a better picture for planners and policy makers. Uttar Pradesh is the fourth largest state with almost 16% of the country's population with nearly 80% of the rural population. Although, the state of Uttar Pradesh has witnessed a decline of MMR from 440 to 216 per 1 lakh live birth from 2004 to 2017, the indicator remains distant from the national average. A survey was done in five selected rural areas of UP, among married women in the age group of 15–49 years, who delivered in the past 15 months to estimate the utilization of health care services. Ninety percent of the total pregnancies were registered. Although, 83% of the women had utilized some of the services, only 5% received full ANC services. 28% pregnant women received 3 antenatal check-ups. A total of 100 IFA tablets were consumed by only 8% of the pregnant women. Nearly 70% of the women had institutional delivery. Although significant number of women had received antenatal care only one-fourth women had received post-natal care.

- Identify the healthcare utilization indicators and comment on the antenatal service utilization in the above scenario
- Compare your findings with the goals mentioned in the National Health Policy (NHP)
- Suggest measures that could be taken to reach the postulated national goal.

Guide Notes

- National Health Policy
- Sustainable Development Goals (SDG)
- *Maternal mortality:* Ratio, rate, direct and indirect causes, and global and national statistics.

EXERCISE 15.2

- At the end of the exercise you should be able to discuss the preventive strategies adopted and the objectives and outcome of the National Tuberculosis Control Program. **(PE34.4)**
- Describe the epidemiology of tuberculosis and its impact on the work, life and economy of India. **(CT1.4)**

National Strategic Plan for TB 2017–2025 was set up by Government of India with a vision of 'TB free India' with zero deaths due to TB. The goal of the programme is to eliminate TB in India by 2025, which is 5 years ahead of the target set by UN Sustainable Development Goals. 50 patients were notified in a DOTS clinic situated in an urbanized village in the month of March 2018. Out of the 50 notified patients, 40 were initiated on the anti-tubercular treatment (ATT) immediately and out of that 30 underwent drug sensitivity testing (DST). On interviewing 10 patients who tested positive for tuberculosis but were not started on ATT, in whom long distances, and time to reach DOTS clinic, longer waiting time, loss of work hours and hence daily wages, were few reasons for the delay or non- initiation of the ATT. 10% of the total new cases registered were put under the defaulter category, before reaching Continuation Phase. 50% of the registered patients received financial support under Nikshay Poshan Yojana.

- Comment on the utilization of health services being provided in the DOTS clinic, in the given scenario.
- Compare your findings with the targets (Outcome indicators), set under National Strategic Plan, 2017–2025.
- Mention the measures taken by the Government of India, in the NSP, 2017–2025 to achieve the above utilization indicators.

Guide Notes

- National Strategic Plan (2017–2025) for TB elimination
- Diagnosis and management of TB
- Drug resistant TB.

EXERCISE 15.3

At the end of the exercise you should be able to enumerate the sources of vital statistics including census, SRS, NFHS, NSSO, etc. **(CM9.7)**

Mission Indradhanush was launched by Government of India in December 2014 to ensure full immunization for children up to two years of age, and pregnant women, with all available vaccines. National Family Health Survey-4 (NFHS-4), conducted in the year 2014–2015, collected data from 29 States and 7 UTs. The data points on immunization coverage in the state of Bihar and West Bengal are as follows:

Bihar

- 62% of children aged 12–23 months received vaccination against six major childhood illnesses.

- 7% have not received any vaccinations at all.
- Dropout from DPT first and third dose was found to be 90–80%, respectively.

West Bengal

- 84% of children aged 12–23 months received all basic vaccinations against six major childhood illnesses (diphtheria, pertussis, tetanus, polio, measles, and tuberculosis).
- 2% have not received any vaccinations at all.
- Dropout between the first and third doses of DPT vaccine from 97 to 93%, respectively.

- Compare the immunization coverage between the two states, i.e. Bihar and West Bengal.
- What could be the possible reasons behind the DPT-3 drop out in the two states?

Guide Notes

- Mission Indradhanush
- Demographical surveys in India with special reference to NFHS-4
- National Immunization Schedule.

EXERCISE 15.4

At the end of the exercise you should be able to describe the age related nutritional needs of infants, children and adolescents including micronutrients and vitamins. **(PE19.1)**

"Global Measles and Rubella Strategic Plan, 2012–2020" was set up with a goal to eliminate Measles in at least 5 of the six WHO regions. India launched one of the world's largest vaccination campaigns on 5th February 2017, against measles, which is a major childhood killer disease, and congenital rubella syndrome responsible for irreversible congenital defects. For the campaign to be effective, it was important that no child is left behind. The MR campaign was introduced in five states of India, namely Goa, Karnataka, Lakshadweep, Puducherry, and Tamil Nadu. In Karnataka a PHC catering to a population of 50000, situated over and around hilly terrain only 550 children received first their dose of MR vaccine.

- Calculate the vaccine coverage of the given PHC.
- Compare your findings with the targets set up by the Measles Elimination Program for the country.

Guide Notes

- Global Vaccine Action Plan and its goals
- Global Measles and Rubella Strategic Plan, 2012–2020
- Primary health centre and services.

EXERCISE 15.5

At the end of the exercise you should be able to enumerate and describe health indicators. **(CM1.7)**

Usually when public health hospitals are evaluated for their efficiency, bed occupancy rates are evaluated. However, the bed occupancy rates are dependent on other variables like length of stay, bed turnover rate (BTR), total number of beds, and total number of admissions and discharges.

Bed turnover rate is calculated by the formula given below:
Bed Turnover Rate (BTR) = Number of discharges (or admissions) in 1 year/active beds.

- Discuss how BTRs will vary in case of different disease conditions (chronic v/s acute diseases)
- In what wards of your hospital do you expect BTR to be on the higher and lower side, respectively. (You might as well go and check the data in the respective wards for validating your assumptions)
- *Which is a better indicator of health:* Quality Adjusted Life Years (QALY) or Health Adjusted Life Expectancy (HALE)? Explain your answer in detail.

Guide Notes

- Mortality and morbidity indicators
- Disability rates
- Indicators of health.

EXERCISE 15.6

At the end of the exercise you should be able to state the vision and outline the goals, strategies and plan of action of NHM and other important national programs pertaining to maternal and child health including RMNCH A+, RBSK, RKSK, JSSK mission Indradhanush and ICDS. **(PE17.1)**

Figure 15.1 shows the trend of maternal mortality ratio (MMR) in the country:

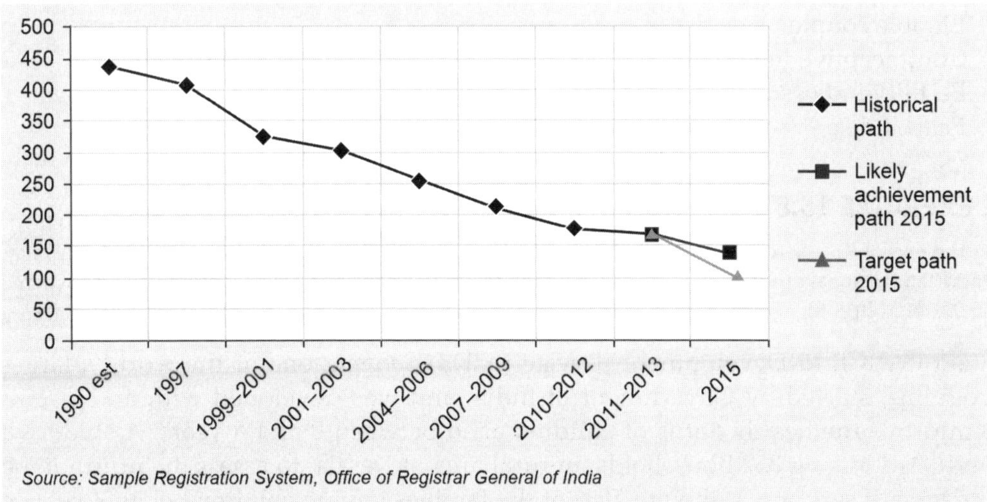

Fig. 15.1: Trends in maternal mortality ratio in India.

- Comment on the utilization of healthcare services provided under RMNCH+A programme in progressing towards the SDG target for MMR of 70 per lakh live births by 2030.
- In a public tertiary care health facility, out of 590 total deliveries in a one-month period, 199 caesarean sections were performed. Calculate and comment on the C-section rate in this healthcare facility.
- What could be the possible reasons behind such a rate?

Guide Notes

- RMNCH+A programme
- Maternal mortality ratio.

EXERCISE 15.7

At the end of the exercise you should be able to state the vision and outline the goals, strategies and plan of action of NHM and other important national programs pertaining to maternal and child health including RMNCH A+, RBSK, RKSK, JSSK mission Indradhanush and ICDS. **(PE17.1)**

In a village of West Bengal with 5000 populations, there are 500 eligible couples. Among these couples, there were 50 married women who had got tubectomy done. 100 eligible women are taking oral contraceptive pills. 50 eligible women are using CuT for family planning. No other means of contraception is used in this village. It is well known that there is no single method of contraception that meets the social, cultural, aesthetic and service needs of all individuals and communities. Keeping this in mind, answer the following.

- What is "Cafeteria Choice"?
- Calculate contraceptive prevalence rate and comment on the finding.
- What are initiatives taken by the Government of India to under RMNCH+A program to address the unmet need for family planning?

Guide Notes

- Family planning
- Eligible couple
- Contraceptive methods
- Fertility indices
- Pearl index.

EXERCISE 15.8

At the end of the exercise you should be able to enumerate and discuss the National Nutrition Policy, important national nutritional Programs including the Integrated Child Development Services Scheme (ICDS), etc. **(CM5.6)**

Integrated Child Development Service (ICDS) Scheme one of the world's largest programs, started by Government of India, and was developed with an objective to improve the health status of children aged between 0 and 6 years. A study was conducted among 352 households, in rural area of Kerala, to assess the utilization of Anganwadi services. Although 70% of the families having children below 3 years of age were utilizing services provided by the Anganwadi centers (AWCs), only 54% of the families with children between 4 and 6 years of age were availing Anganwadi services. Only 2 out of 193 women in reproductive age group (19–44 years) utilized ICDS services.

- Comment on the utilization of services provided by the Anganwadi centers in the above scenario.
- What measures can be taken at various levels by the government to improve the utilization of the same?

Guide Notes

- Integrated Child Development Service (ICDS) Scheme.
- Functions and services provided by an Anganwadi worker (AWW).

EXERCISE 15.9

At the end of the exercise you should be able to demonstrate infection control practices and use of personal protective equipment (PPE). **(MI8.7)**

Sheena has been suffering from fever and burning micturition, on and off, for over a month, for which she took medicines from a nearby pharmacy. The pharmacy handed her antibiotics along with antipyretics, which she would take only for as long as her symptoms lasted. She was counselled by one of her friends to see a doctor since her symptoms are recurring. On consulting a doctor, Sheena was asked to get urine culture test done along with several other investigations. Meanwhile she was given symptomatic treatment, which she took for 3 days and when her symptoms improved, she forgot to follow-up with the doctor. After two weeks, she again developed similar symptoms and was rushed to the doctor along with her test reports. The doctor told Sheena that her reports showed that she has urinary tract infection (UTI) and has also developed resistance to few antibiotics commonly used to treat UTI.

- What do you think are the common reasons for development of antimicrobial resistance (AMR) in our country?
- What are the goals and objectives of National Action Plan for curbing the development of AMR?
- What are the focus areas of National Action Plan for antimicrobial resistance strategic priorities?

Guide Notes

- Antimicrobial resistance (AMR).
- National Action Plan–Antimicrobial resistance.

EXERCISE 15.10

At the end of the exercise you should be able to educate health care workers on national programs of tuberculosis and administering and monitoring the DOTS program. **(CT1.18)**

Radha, an ASHA of a small village of Katihar district (Bihar), on her routine visit to the village found that Mr Mahesh was bedridden, and his TB symptoms have worsened. Three months back, Radha had taken him to District Microscopy Centre for his long-standing cough and after his diagnosis was confirmed as TB, he was started DOTS. On enquiring with his family, Radha found that Mahesh had stopped taking treatment as he was experiencing some side-effects. His neighbours, thereafter, convinced him that the treatment is dangerous and lifelong and that he won't be able to resume his work if he continued the treatment. Radha called her ANM *didi*, Savita who was a trained treatment supporter. Savita counselled Mahesh and explained to him the consequences of abruptly stopping the treatment. Mahesh was then started on MDR-TB drug regimen and is currently adhering to his treatment.

- What are the important reasons for non-compliance to DOTS?
- What are the major causes of out-of-pocket expenditure (OOPE) in TB patients?
- How can adherence to TB treatment be improved?
- What are the strategic pillars of National Strategic Plan for TB elimination?

Guide Notes

- Tuberculosis
- DOTS and DOTS plus
- National Strategic Plan for TB elimination (2017–25).

EXERCISE 15.15

- At the end of the exercise you should be able to describe various methods of treatment of hospital waste. **(CM14.2)**
- Describe laws related to hospital waste management. **(CM14.3)**

Rinki Devi was ANM at Health and Wellness Centre (HWC) Ratanpur (Chhattisgarh). After population enumeration and completion of community-based assessment checklist, with the help of ASHA, she organized NCD screening. During the screening, Mr. Jatin was found to be obese and had high blood glucose level on testing with glucometer. He was referred to the concerned PHC, where the medical officer diagnosed him with diabetes. He received his medications as well as advises on lifestyle modifications. During her monthly follow-up visit, Rinki Devi found that Mr Jatin was not adhering to the advice given to him for lifestyle modification and was also non-compliant to his medications. She counselled him about following a healthy diet, including physical exercises in his routine, avoiding tobacco and alcohol, adhering to the treatment and about long- and short-term complications of diabetes. Jatin told Rinki Devi that he was aware of these measures, but it has been difficult for him to follow them due to time constraint and limited availability of healthy food options.

- Mention the facilities provided at an HWC.
- What are the various factors for poor adherence to lifestyle modifications to control NCDs?
- How can we improve compliance to lifestyle modifications?

Guide Notes

- Lifestyle Modification
- National Programme for Prevention and Control of Cancer, Diabetes, Cardiovascular Diseases and Stroke (NPCDCS)
- *AB-HWC:* One of the subcomponents of Ayushman Bharat Scheme by GOI.

EXERCISE 15.16

At the end of the exercise you should be able to describe and discuss the following National Health programs including immunization, tuberculosis, leprosy, malaria, HIV, filaria, kala azar, diarrheal diseases, anemia and nutritional disorders, blindness, non-communicable diseases, cancer and iodine deficiency. **(PH1.55)**

Few of the educational institutions in the city were assessed for compliance with COTPA (Cigarettes and Other Tobacco Products Act). It was observed that most of the schools were not displaying signboards for 'No Tobacco Use' within 100 yards of their premises. Also, tobacco vendors were present within 100 yards of the institutions and signs of tobacco use within campus were found.

- What constitutes violation of Section 6 of COTPA Act and what is the fine for the same?
- What are the main barriers to successful implementation of COTPA?
- How will you carry out awareness programme for tobacco control in schools?

Guide Notes

- Cigarettes and Other Tobacco Products Act

- National Tobacco Control Programme (NTCP)
- School Awareness Programme for Tobacco Control
- Smokeless tobacco.

EXERCISE 15.17

At the end of the exercise you should be able to demonstrate awareness about laws pertaining to practice of medicine such as clinical establishment act and Human Organ Transplantation Act and its implications. **(CM20.4)**

A raid was carried out at a nursing home in Haryana after complaints regarding illegal ultrasonography were registered against it. The nursing home was being run by a doctor with BAMS degree and no radiologist was registered with the nursing home. Form-F having patients' details and reasons for conducting sonography, which was required to be filled in completely and sent timely to the Appropriate Authority was incomplete and were not being sent regularly. The date and the signature of the doctor were also missing on the forms. Many aberrations were observed at the nursing home and hence suspension of registration of the sonography machine and sealing of the equipment were carried out.

- What constitutes violation of PC-PNDT act?
- What is the responsibility of medical professional towards PC-PNDT act?
- What are the functions of Appropriate Authority under PC-PNDT Act?

Guide Notes

- Form-F while conducting an Ultrasonography during ANC visits of a pregnant female
- PC-PNDT Act
- Violations and Appropriate Authority.

EXERCISE 15.18

- At the end of the exercise you should be able to enumerate the contraceptive methods for male and female. Discuss their advantages and disadvantages. **(PY9.6)**
- Counsel in a simulated environment, contraception and puerperal sterilization. **(OG19.2)**
- Describe and discuss the temporary and permanent methods of contraception, indications, technique and complications; selection of patients, side effects and failure rate including OC, male contraception, emergency contraception and IUCD. **(OG 21.1)**

Reena and her husband, a newly married couple, plans on having their first child after 2 years of marriage. Her friend suggested her to consult the doctor at her nearby PHC, where she was prescribed combined oral contraceptive pills (OCPs) for contraception, after careful history taking and clinical examination. Six months later, Reena presented herself to the PHC complaining about missed periods. Sujata who is the ANM at the PHC enquired about the OCPs, to which Reena said that she had not been regular with the medicines as she was having side effects or sometimes, she would just forget to take them. Her urine pregnancy test (UPT) was found to be negative. Reena was then counseled by Sujata about taking her birth control pills (BCPs) regularly and to report to the PHC if she develops any serious side effects.

- What are the barriers to contraceptive needs?
- How will you improve compliance to OCPs?
- What are the guidelines to be followed in case of missed pills?

Guide Notes

- Contraceptive need
- Oral contraceptive pills
- Management of missed pill.

EXERCISE 15.19

At the end of the exercise you should be able to describe food hygiene. **(CM5.7)**

Based on checklist stipulated by Food Safety and Standards Authority of India (FSSAI), inspection of few slaughter houses of Hanumanthuwaka in Visakhapatnam was carried out by food safety officers to identify the level of compliance. It was found that few slaughterhouses did not have provision for hot water in slaughter room, ante mortem or postmortem examination was not being carried out as per the specified proforma, no separate space for segregation and storage of carcasses were present, and no record of food handler's medical examination and no record of products were being maintained. The regulator issued notices, expecting improvements, to the slaughterhouses, failure to comply with which will lead to shutting down of those slaughterhouses.

- What are the main functions of FSSAI?
- What are the personal hygiene requirements of food handlers/employees?
- What is the purpose of ante mortem and postmortem examination?

Guide Notes

- Food safety and standards act, 2006; compare with PFA act 1954
- Slaughterhouse sanitation guidelines
- Food handler's hygiene guidelines.

EXERCISE 15.20

- At the end of the exercise you should be able to Define and describe the concept of international health. **(CM18.1)**
- Describe roles of various international health agencies. **(CM18.2)**

A pregnant woman was admitted to a medical college in Gujarat with complaint of low-grade fever. She did not have any history of travel in the last three months. Her blood sample was tested at the medical college for dengue, after which she was provisionally found positive for the Zika virus. Her serum sample was sent to the National Institute of Virology (NIV), Pune where it was confirmed to be Zika virus positive. She delivered an apparently healthy baby who did not exhibit any markers of microcephaly. The same was notified to National Centre for Disease Control (NCDC), which would further notify WHO under International Health Regulations.

- What are the deciding criteria to notify public health events under International Health Regulations?
- What are the principles of International Health Regulations?
- How can compliance to IHR be assessed?

Guide Notes

- International Health Regulations (2005)

- Public Health Emergency of International Concern
- Core capacities
- GOARN.

EXERCISE 15.21

- At the end of the exercise you should be able to describe the role, benefits and functioning of the Employee's State Insurance Scheme. **(CM11.2)**
- Enumerate and describe specific occupational health hazards, their risk factors and preventive measures. **(CM11.3)**

A 75-year-old male patient presents to the emergency department of tertiary care hospital with a dry cough and shortness of breath. Patient has been experiencing shortness of breath for 2 months and dry cough persisting for nearly 6 months. Patient reports feeling breathless and sometimes temporarily unable to breathe when at rest and especially when walking up the stairs. Additionally, he reports having an unexplained weight loss in the last 6 months. Patient is a non-smoker and has a history of high BP which has been under control for years with medication. When asked about his occupation, he reported that he had worked for almost 30years in a shipyard, and has retired over time. On examination it is seen that there is clubbing in his fingers, but cannot ascertain when it began. Further there is a crackling sound heard on auscultation of his lungs. His chest X-ray shows irregular opacities in his lungs and there is evidence of non-calcified pleural plaque.

- What is the provisional diagnosis of this case with reasons?
- What may be the differential diagnosis?
- What further investigation is needed to reach to the final diagnosis?
- What is pneumoconiosis? What are the various types of pneumoconiosis and their associated risk factors?
- How can pneumoconiosis be treated and prevented?
- What benefits under the ESI Act is the patient eligible for?

Guide Notes

- Occupational health laws and provisions regulating the health of workers in an establishment
- ESI Act, 1948.

REFERENCES

1. Kadri's IAPSM's Textbook of Community Medicine. 2nd edn, pages 144, 203, 205, 238, 254, 285, 312, 317, 368, 464, 473, 566, 609, 626, 695, 720, 722, 724, 753, 777, 784, 817, 864-866,876, 884, 906, 919, 925, 934, 940, 954, 984
2. Park's Textbook of Preventive and Social Medicine. 26th edn, pages 464, 552, 964.

FURTHER READING

1. Bio-Medical Waste Management Rules 2016, Ministry of environment, forest and climate Change, Government of India.http://moef.gov.in/wp-content/uploads/2019/10/BMW-Rules- 2016_1-4.pdf
2. Food Safety and Standards Act 2006, Available fromhttps://fssai.gov.in/upload/uploadfiles/files/FOOD-ACT.pdf

3. Gazette of India. The Pre-Conception and Pre-Natal Diagnostic Techniques (Prohibition of Sex Selection) Act, 1994 (At No.57 of 1994) [As amended by Prenatal diagnostic Techniques (Regulation and prevention of misuse) Act,2002].
4. Government of India. Ministry of Health and Family Welfare. National Programme for Prevention and Control of Cancer, Diabetes, Cardiovascular Diseases and Stroke (NPCDCS). Operational Guidelines; 2013-2017
5. International Health Regulations (2005). Geneva: World Health Organization; 2005. Available from: http://apps.who.int/iris/bitstream/10665/246107/1/9789241580496-eng.pdf
6. International Health Regulations. (2005). IHR core capacity monitoring framework: questionnaire for monitoring progress in the implementation of IHR core capacities in States Parties. 2017 Questionnaire. Geneva: World Health Organization 2017. Available from http://apps.who.int/iris/bitstream/10665/255756/1/WHO-WHE-CPI-2017.41-eng.pdf
7. Laxminarayan R, Chaudhury RR (2016) Antibiotic Resistance in India: Drivers and Opportunities for Action. PLoS Med 13(3): e1001974.
8. Ministry of Health and Family Welfare, Government of India. Handbook of PCPNDT Act and Rules with Amendments. New Delhi: 2006. Available from: http://www.iria.in/uploadNotices/Handbook_on_PNDT_Act.pdf
9. Ministry of Health and Family Welfare, Government of India, National Multi-sectoral Action Plan for Prevention and Control of Non-communicable Diseases (2017-22)
10. National Action Plan on Antimicrobial Resistance (NAP-AMR) [Internet] http://www.searo.who.int/india/topics/antimicrobial_resistance/nap_amr.pdf
11. National Cold Chain Vaccine Management Resource Center, National Institute of Health and Family Welfare. National Effective Vaccine Management Assessment, India 2013. New Delhi, India: Ministry of Health and Family Welfare; 2013.
12. Resource Package for Quality Improvement cycles in LaQshya, GOI, Maternal Health Division, November 2018
13. The Cigarettes and Other Tobacco Products (Prohibition of Advertisement and regulation of Trade and Commerce, Production, Supply and Distribution) Act, 2003; An Act Enacted by the Parliament of Republic of India by Notification in the Official Gazette.
14. World Health Organization. Effective Vaccine Management (EVM) Initiative, EVM Assessment Tools and User Guides, the EVM Site Selection Tool. Immunization, Vaccines and Biologicals. Geneva, Switzerland: World Health Organization; 2010. Available from: http://www.who.int/immunization/programmes_systems/supply_chain/evm/en/index3.html.

CHAPTER

16

Health Ethics

Competency code	Competency addressed	Exercise
CM6.2	Describe and discuss the principles and demonstrate the methods of collection, classification, analysis, interpretation and presentation of statistical data	16.1–16.10

EXERCISE 16.1

At the end of this exercise, you should be able to describe and discuss the principles and demonstrate the methods of collection, classification, analysis, interpretation and presentation of statistical data. **(CM6.2)**

Dr Abhi is a practicing pediatrician in Delhi who was convinced by the current research published in medical journals and decided to treat the pediatric malaria patients with a drug 'X'. Drug X is currently approved for treatment of other diseases but not for malaria in India. Dr Bijoy planned to give a Drug 'Y' to the pediatric malaria cases coming to his clinic. Y is a newly approved drug for pediatric malaria in India. Dr Chinmaya who is also a practicing pediatrician in the same region is willing to give Drug 'Z' to the pediatric patients reporting to his clinic with malaria. Drug Z is currently approved for treatment of malaria in adults but not in pediatric cases in India.

- Which of the above cases is/are clinical trial and which is/are clinical practice and why?
- What is the basic difference between clinical trial and clinical practice?

Guide Notes

- Various reports on medical ethical issues
- RCT and types of RCTs.

Exercise 16.2

At the end of this exercise, you should be able to describe and discuss the principles and demonstrate the methods of collection, classification, analysis, interpretation and presentation of statistical data. **(CM6.2)**

You are one of the members of the Institutional Ethics Committee (IEC) of your Institute. The Ethics committee comprises of a total of 10 members, 7 members from your institute including four clinicians, two basic scientists, you as the member secretary and

3 members unassociated with your institute; two social scientists and one lawyer. In the last 2 months, a total of 46 protocols were submitted to the IEC for approval. On the day of the IEC meeting, it was found that only 3 members of the Ethics committee are present. But the Chairman of the Ethics Committee decides to continue with the meeting, where after the attending members approved 20 proposals.

- Is there any problem associated with ethics committee composition?
- According to ICMR guidelines, what are the requirements for being the member of the Ethics Committee?
- Was it appropriate to approve the protocol in the presence of only three members? State the reason for the same.

Guide Note

- ICMR Guidelines for approval of protocol for conducting research.

EXERCISE 16.3

At the end of this exercise, you should be able to describe and discuss the principles and demonstrate the methods of collection, classification, analysis, interpretation and presentation of statistical data. **(CM 6.2)**

In 1932, US Public Health Division conducted a study related to epidemiology of syphilis among the male population of the Macon County, Alabama. This was an observational study including 399 men with syphilis and 201 men without syphilis and they all were followed for 40 years, i.e. till 1972.

During the study, researchers posing as physicians informed the study subjects already infected with syphilis that they were going to receive treatment for "Bad Blood" (a then locally used term for syphilis). Contrary to reality, none of the patients received any kind of treatment. Consequently in 1972, one Public Health Service (PHS), Sexually Transmitted Diseases (STD) investigator Peter Buxton, went to press with allegations of gross ethical violations by the aforementioned research group.

- Which ethical principles were violated in this study?
- What was the main guiding ethical principles described in Belmonte report?

Guide Notes

- Belmont report
- Ethical principles.

EXERCISE 16.4

At the end of this exercise, you should be able to describe and discuss the principles and demonstrate the methods of collection, classification, analysis, interpretation and presentation of statistical data. **(CM6.2)**

In the years 1946–48, after World war II "Orvus-mapharsen", one of the least known experiments in the history of research; details of which had been kept a secret for almost six decades, was conducted. Before the said study, there were reports about the effectiveness of Post Exposure Prophylaxis in animals who had syphilis.US-Public Health Services (US-PHS) then, was interested in knowing whether the solution would be effective in humans. As already known, establishing efficacy required controlled intentional exposure of the research subject, preferably via natural methods such as sexual intercourse, the researchers exposed Prisoners of War (PoW) to syphilis through sexual intercourse with commercial sex workers (CSWs) already carrying the disease. During this period, commercial sex work was legal in Guatemala. Other vulnerable populations such are soldiers and psychiatric patients were also included in this study. They also tried an invasive method where syphilitic emulsions were applied after intentionally producing abrasions on subjects' genitals. No informed consent was taken during this study.

- Which ethical principles were violated in this study?

Guide Notes

- Violation of ethical principles
- Types of consent
- Composition of a research group
- GCP guidelines.

EXERCISE 16.5

At the end of this exercise, you should be able to describe and discuss the principles and demonstrate the methods of collection, classification, analysis, interpretation and presentation of statistical data. **(CM6.2)**

Researchers want to test a new drug X for the treatment of malaria in children, and simultaneously want to compare its efficacy with one established drug Y. In a previous trial, it was reported that drug X was less efficacious than Y and had side-effects like drowsiness and development of rash. Researchers thought these were mild symptoms and did not inform the same to the parents before enrolling their children in the study. However, consent form was signed by either parents, and the child was enrolled into the study.

- What ethical problems do you see with this study?
- Is it required to take consent from both the parents, or approval of either parent is sufficient for enrollment of their ward?
- What are the different types of assent, based on age group?
  After obtaining the ethical clearance, the researchers found that they forgot to include the demographic, socioeconomic status, and previous history of malaria in the approved protocol and hence had to re-apply for it, but until then decided to continue the study.
- Explain whether it is ethical to collect the data not mentioned in the approved protocol?

Guide Notes

- Difference between assent and consent
- Procedure to be followed while re-applying for ethical approval
- IRB and its members.

EXERCISE 16.6

At the end of this exercise, you should be able to describe and discuss the principles and demonstrate the methods of collection, classification, analysis, interpretation and presentation of statistical data. **(CM6.2)**

You are posted as a Medical Officer In-charge of a primary health care (PHC) centre. In a monthly supervisory meeting, one of your health workers (HWs) reported a dropout case of immunization from the last session. The HW further informed that on visiting their house, the family denied immunizing their second child, because of development of seizure following immunization in the first child. You, also being the District Immunization Officer (DIO), visited the house, but the family is still unwilling to get the child vaccinated.

- Can the child be immunized against the parent's will?
- Which ethical principles will be violated if they are vaccinated forcefully?

Guide Notes

- Role of DIO in the routine immunization of a child within the district
- Ethical issues during a drug trial or vaccination drive.

EXERCISE 16.7

At the end of this exercise, you should be able to describe and discuss the principles and demonstrate the methods of collection, classification, analysis, interpretation and presentation of statistical data. **(CM 6.2)**

A pharmaceutical company is interested in testing a new drug for managing gallbladder carcinoma (Ca GB). The drug is expected to increase survival by 1.8 years without any significant side effects, except for nausea and vomiting, which is reported to occur within 24 hours of chemotherapy. In one year, a single cycle of chemotherapy is required to show the expected results. One of the Principal Investigator (PI) for this study is from your institute and has submitted the protocol to the Ethics Committee. According to the protocol, during the study, consent was taken from the participants. The company decides to award 300 USD to the participants, for each dose of chemotherapy they take. All the participants will be followed up for a period of 3 years, during which they will receive the drug free of any cost. However, the protocol stays unvoiced about the definite treatment of the survivors. As a part of the Ethics Committee of the institute, you receive the protocol for review.

- What is/are the ethical problem(s) associated with this study?
- Which ethical guidelines clarify this issue?

Guide Notes

- Role of ethics committee of an institute
- Ethical guidelines to conduct any research involving live human subjects.
- HSP/PHRP certification.

EXERCISE 16.8

At the end of this exercise, you should be able to describe and discuss the principles and demonstrate the methods of collection, classification, analysis, interpretation and presentation of statistical data. **(CM 6.2)**

You are a member of the Ethics Committee of your Institute. A research proposal came to you for review. A researcher wants to test a new drug 'X5331' for treatment of moderate anemia in adolescent girls. Currently, oral ferrous sulphate is the approved treatment of moderate anemia in India under Anemia Mukt Bharat Initiative. The researcher plans to divide the study subjects into two groups, one group will receive the drug of interest along with dietary counselling, while the other group will receive a placebo with dietary counselling. The placebo was designed in such a way that it resembles the drug X5331 in every aspect. Blood samples will be collected serially after intervals of 6 weeks, for a total period of 6 months, to evaluate the levels of serum ferritin, transferrin, and hemoglobin in both the groups. The researcher has submitted the documents required (protocol, consent form, participant information sheet in local language) for obtaining approval and has made it clear in the protocol that consent will be duly taken by the participants.

- Do you identify any ethical problems in this study? Why?
- If the study is ethically correct, then what other documents do the researcher need to submit before commencing the study?

Guide Notes

- Role of placebo in medical research
- Blinding and its type
- Responsible conduct of research (RCR) certification.

EXERCISE 16.9

At the end of this exercise, you should be able to describe and discuss the principles and demonstrate the methods of collection, classification, analysis, interpretation and presentation of statistical data. **(CM 6.2)**

The drug 'A' is already approved for managing bipolar disorder (BPD) in India. A research team who planned to test this drug 'A' for treatment of schizophrenia against the drug 'B' which is already approved for the disease, was given clearance from the Ethics Committee. The primary objective is to study the role of the drug 'A' on various neurochemical, i.e. serotonin, dopamine, etc. The study was started on a group of patients presenting to the clinic only after a written consent form had been signed by both the participant and the researcher. Two blood samples, each 5 ml, were collected from the participants, one at the beginning of the study and the other, 6 weeks after initiation of the drug under research.

- What is/are the ethical issue(s) associated with this study?
- Since the drug is already approved for some other condition, do these researchers need fresh CTRI registration for their study related to schizophrenia?
- After the study was over the team decided to analyze other blood parameters namely complete blood count (CBC) and serum urea and creatinine to find whether there is any effect of drug 'A' on these parameters too. Comment on whether fresh ethical approval and consent are required for this analysis or not?

Guide Note

- Registration of clinical trial.

EXERCISE 16.10

At the end of this exercise, you should be able to describe and discuss the principles and demonstrate the methods of collection, classification, analysis, interpretation and presentation of statistical data. **(CM 6.2)**

A study was being planned to compare a new drug 'X' with iron sucrose, used for treatment of anemia. The study was duly approved by the ethics committee for two years and consent was taken from the participants during the study. In the interim report submitted to the ethics committee it was found that there was no statistically significant difference between the results obtained on using the drug 'X' and Iron sucrose. Additionally, subjects put on drug 'X' developed diarrhea and vomiting.

- Being a member of the Ethics Committee, decide whether you should allow the study to continue till completion?
- Out of the 20 study subjects, 10 patients developed severe diarrhea, and were therefore admitted to the hospital, where later 6 patients succumbed to death. With this data what is your impression about continuation of the study?
- What are the different types of serious adverse events that must be reported?

Guide Notes

- Open label trials
- Superiority, equivalence and non-inferiority trials
- SAE and AE (adverse events) in human drug trials.

REFERENCES

1. Kadri's IAPSM's Textbook of Community Medicine. 2nd edn, page 194.
2. Park's Textbook of Preventive and Social Medicine. 26th edn, page 92.

FURTHER READING

1. Belmont Report, Available at: https://www.hhs.gov/ohrp/sites/default/files/the-belmont-report-508c_FINAL.pdf.
2. Declaration of Helsinki ethical principles for medical research involving human subjects. Available at: https://www.wma.net/policies-post/wma-declaration-of-helsinki-ethical-principles-for-medical-research-involving-human-subjects/
3. Handbook National Ethical Guidelines for Biomedical and Health Research Involving Human Participants, Indian Council of Medical Research, 2018.
4. National Ethical Guidelines, Indian Council of Medical Research, Available at: https://ethics.ncdirindia.org//asset/pdf/ICMR_National_Ethical_Guidelines.pdf.
5. National Ethical Guidelines for Biomedical Research Involving Children, Indian Council of Medical Research , New Delhi, 2017, Available at: https://main.icmr.nic.in/sites/default/files/guidelines/ National_Ethical_Guidelines_for_BioMedic al_Research_Involving_Children_0.pdf.
6. Serious Adverse Events, Central Drug Standards Control Organization, Govt. of India. Available at: https://cdsco.gov.in/opencms/opencms/en/Clinical-Trial/SAE/
7. Tuskegee Study, Available at: https://www.cdc.gov/tuskegee/index.html.
8. World Health Organization, Casebook on ethical issues in international health research.

Index